OXFORD MEDICAL PUBLICATIONS

Zeis' Manual of Plastic Surgery

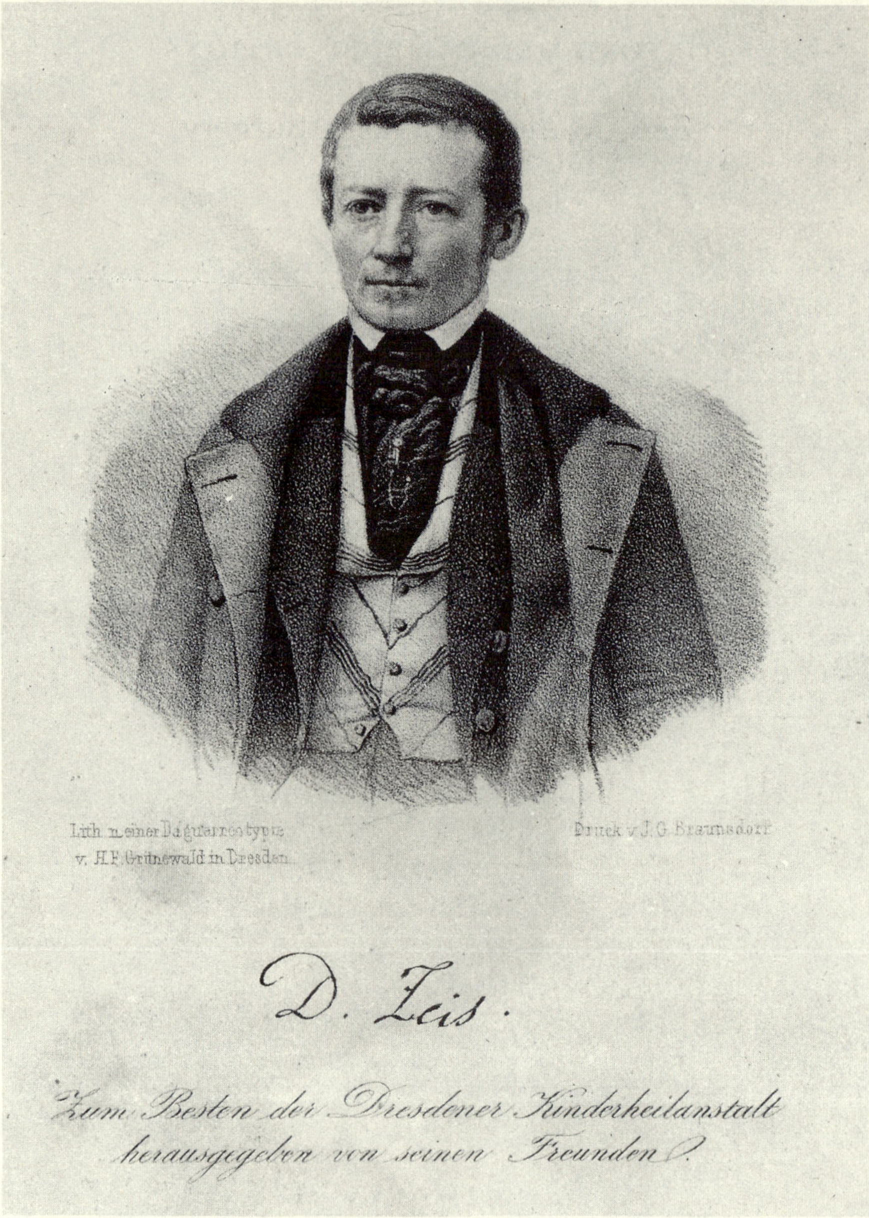

Eduard Zeis (1807–1868). The portrait is dated 'c.1842'; the signature is lithographed, and the 'D' is an abbreviation for 'Doctor'. (Reproduced by kind permission of the Department of Prints and Drawings of the Zentralbibliothek, Zürich.)

ZEIS' MANUAL
of
PLASTIC SURGERY

Translated from:

Handbuch der plastischen Chirurgie
von Eduard Zeis

Berlin 1838

by

T. J. S. PATTERSON MD, M.Chir., FRCS

Blair O. Rogers Research Fellow in the History of Plastic Surgery, Wellcome Unit for the History of Medicine, Oxford

Oxford New York Tokyo
OXFORD UNIVERSITY PRESS
1988

Oxford University Press, Walton Street, Oxford OX2 6DP
Oxford New York Toronto
Delhi Bombay Calcutta Madras Karachi
Petaling Jaya Singapore Hong Kong Tokyo
Nairobi Dar es Salaam Cape Town
Melbourne Auckland
and associated companies in
Berlin Ibadan

Oxford is a trade mark of Oxford University Press

Published in the United States
by Oxford University Press, New York

Handbuch der plastischen Chirurgie
first published in German by G. Reimer, Berlin, 1838. English translation first published 1988.

British Library Cataloguing in Publication Data
Zeis, Edward, 1807–1868
Zeis' manual of plastic surgery.
1. Medicine. Plastic surgery
I. Title II. Handbuck der plastischen
Chirurgie. English
617'.95
ISBN 0-19-261746-X

Library of Congress Cataloging in Publication Data
Zeis, Eduard.
Zeis' manual of plastic surgery.
(Oxford medical publications)
"Translated from Handbuch der plastischen Chirurgie
von Eduard Zeis, Berlin 1838."
Includes bibliographical references and index.
1. Surgery, Plastic—Handbooks, manuals, etc.—
Early works to 1900. I. Patterson, Thomas J. S.
(Thomas John Starling) II. Title. III. Title: Manual
of plastic surgery. IV. Series. [DNLM: 1. Surgery,
Plastic. WO 600 Z4h]
RD118.Z4513 1988 617'.95 88-9983
ISBN 0-19-261746-X

Typesetting by Computerised Typesetting Services Limited,
Redhill, Surrey.
Printed in Great Britain
at the University Printing House, Oxford
by David Stanford,
Printer to the University

CONTENTS

TRANSLATOR'S INTRODUCTION

Eduard Zeis, in his *Manual* in 1838, introduced the term 'plastic surgery' for a branch of surgery that was developing rapidly in the first half of the nineteenth century. When the book was reviewed in London in 1839, the reviewer knew of only four authors who had written on the subject: Zeis in Dresden, Blandin in Paris, Dieffenbach in Berlin, and Liston in Edinburgh and London.[1] Only the first two had attempted to cover the whole field, and the reviewer gave most of his attention to them. In spite of some criticisms, Zeis' book, when compared with Blandin's, was shown to be 'unquestionably the more perfect and better arranged'. Thus it can be regarded as the first textbook of plastic surgery. It has not previously been translated into English.

At the beginning of the nineteenth century plastic surgery was not part of surgical practice. Tagliacozzi's detailed instructions for the restoration of noses and lips, by skin from the arm, were almost forgotten. After his death in 1599 very few surgeons attempted to copy his operations, which were generally misunderstood or recalled in ribald and contemptuous terms. The news from India at the end of the eighteenth century, that noses and lips could be reconstructed with skin from the forehead, re-awakened interest in Europe, and, in 1816, Carpue in London and von Gräfe in Berlin showed that the classical Indian and Italian operations were still practicable.

Zeis was a general surgeon, with an interest in ophthalmology and the diseases of children. His special interest in plastic surgery was inspired by Dieffenbach,[2] who had begun to devote more and more time to it from about 1828. Dieffenbach's originality in the design of new operations, and his boldness in carrying them out, made him the leading figure in the specialty until his death in 1847. Zeis was some-

[1] On plastic surgery, *Br. for. med. Rev.* **7**, 386 (1839).

[2] Johann Friedrich Dieffenbach (1792–1847) was director of the surgical department at the Charité in Berlin (1829), and professor (1832). He succeeded von Gräfe as director of the university surgical clinic in 1840. After his death in 1847 his place was taken by Bernhard Langenbeck (1810–87). For a biography of Dieffenbach see: R. M. Goldwyn, Johann Friedrich Dieffenbach, *Plastic reconstr. Surg.* **42**, 18 (1968).

times criticized for his lavish praise of Dieffenbach,[3] with the implication that he did this because he had been one of his pupils. But Zeis made it clear that he had never been a pupil of Dieffenbach's, and that he was under no particular obligation to him. He only gave him the honour that he deserved, for his services to plastic surgery were greater than those of any other surgeon. Zeis himself did not make any major contributions to operative surgery, but he was an experienced and skilful surgeon who was competent to evaluate the new techniques as they were being developed. He was a prolific writer, publishing a large number of papers on diverse surgical subjects, but his passion was to collect material relating to plastic operations and their history. He is now remembered for his writings on plastic surgery.

He had been taught by von Ammon and von Walther that surgery and medicine should be brought closer together, and that surgery should be based on physiology. He emphasized these principles in his book: the importance of the general condition of the patient, including the mental state, on the outcome of the operation, and the need to identify and eradicate any underlying disease (particularly in view of the prevalence of syphilis and the effects of its over-treatment with mercury). He devoted a separate chapter to the physiology of skin flaps, with the changes during and after transplantation, the conditions necessary for primary healing, and the problems of infection and contraction. He was keen to point out the benefits of plastic surgery, not only for improving appearance, but also for restoring function—returning disfigured patients to normal human company, and enabling them to earn a living. But he took a realistic view of its limitations. Since skin alone was used for reconstruction, the reconstructed part was bound to differ from normal, mainly because of lack of supporting tissues. He was always prepared to point out the failures and the areas where further advances were needed, but he found it hard to define the boundaries of this new speciality. The criterion was to be 'transplantation of tissue' (primarily skin). This led him to exclude simple repair of congenital clefts of the lip and palate. But he included tenotomy because he was particularly interested in it. He recognized the importance of Dupuytren's work on contracture of the palmar fascia, and he gave a full account of this at a time when little was known about it in Germany.

---

[3] '. . . even more than the ordinary allowance of flattery, which, however merited, must, in such doses, be rather nauseating to the Berlin professor'. *Br. for. med. Rev.* **7**, 408 (1839).

For the transplantation of skin, the simpler and more certain Indian method soon came to be preferred to the arduous Italian method. All attention was then directed to the design of other local flaps. Free grafts were not thought to be reliable enough for routine use—the few experiments and clinical attempts had mostly been a failure, and the occasional reunion of completely separated pieces of tissue, although always of interest to surgeons, was still not well understood. But local flaps found many applications—at first to the repair of defects of the nose and lips, then to the eyelids and other parts of the face, and then to other parts of the body to help with general surgical problems, such as fistulas of the genitourinary system and intestines, and the repair of hernias. After the excision of tumours, as of the lip and the breast, repair with flaps gave more rapid healing and relief of disability.

Zeis described the necessary operative techniques in great detail, often illustrated by diagrams and case reports, with the indications, complications, and the secondary corrections that might be needed. He believed that specialization was the key to improvement in surgical treatment, and he hoped that his book would provide the basis for this, and encourage more surgeons to attempt plastic operations.

BIOGRAPHY OF EDUARD ZEIS (1807–68)

Eduard Zeis was born in Dresden on 1 October 1807, the son of a rich business man. In 1827 he started his medical studies at Leipzig University. His father suffered a major financial disaster at this time, which would have made his son's further studies impossible if a wealthy relative had not helped him. In 1829 he went to Bonn, where he became a pupil of von Walther,[4] and was so impressed by him that he followed him to Munich when he became professor there. Von Walther appointed Zeis as his assistant, and became the guiding star in his life. Zeis often recalled his old teacher with touching, almost child-like affection.

In 1830 he returned to Leipzig as assistant to the surgeon,

[4] Phillipp Franz von Walther (1782–1849), professor of physiology and surgery at Landshut (1804), with a particular interest in surgery and ophthalmology, did much to bring surgery, medicine, and physiology together, demanding the full medical training for surgeons, rather than the more practical training that had been carried out up till then. From 1818–30 he was in Bonn as professor of surgery, and, with von Gräfe, started (1820) the *Journal der Chirurgie und Augenheilkunde*, in which many of the early papers on plastic surgery were published. From 1830 he was professor in Munich and personal physician to King Ludwig I.

Kohlrusch, completing his medical studies, and graduating on 22 June 1832 with a dissertation on *Herniae cruralis externae historia cum epicrisi*.[5] He then went back to Dresden in practice, with a particular interest in surgery, diseases of the eye, and diseases of children. He joined three other doctors in founding the Children's Hospital, and played a major part in the formation of the Dresden Medical Society, which was soon involved in the debates on medical reform in Saxony. Throughout this period he was supported by von Ammon,[6] who encouraged his interest in diseases of the eye. This led him to investigate the glands of the eyelid. He established the relation of the Meibomian glands to the hairs and the diseases of the hair follicles, and showed the difference between infection of a sebaceous gland and distension of a Meibomian gland. The sebaceous glands in the free borders of the eyelids are still known as the 'glands of Zeis'.

In 1844 he was appointed professor of surgery and director of the surgical clinic in Marburg, with a testimonial from von Ammon, which included, among many tributes to his skills as a surgeon and a writer, the information that he was a competent Latinist, and spoke Spanish, English, and French, and was planning to write a history of surgery. The salary was less than he was getting in Dresden, but he gladly accepted a post that brought him a chair in an academic department of surgery. He soon found that, coming from a big city, he was regarded as a foreigner in the narrow provincialism of Marburg. From the moment of his inauguration he was involved in intrigue and quarrels with his colleagues, which continued until he resigned in 1850 to return to Dresden. He had succeeded Christoph Ullmann, who was a poor surgeon and teacher. Much of the surgical work had been done by Bünger, the professor of anatomy, and by H. L. F. Robert, the assistant professor of surgery. Robert was a true child of Marburg—his grandfather had been professor of theology, his father had been vice-chancellor, and his sister was married to Heusinger, the professor of medicine. Through the influence of his father, Robert had been appointed assistant professor, against the wishes of the university, at a very young age. Before Zeis arived he had taken over more and more of the surgery and the teaching from Ullmann, and he had expected to get the chair. He made vigorous efforts to discredit Zeis with the authorities and the students. He opened a private clinic, which attracted patients and

[5] History and diagnosis of femoral hernia.

[6] Friedrich August von Ammon (1799–1861)—surgeon and professor (1828) in Dresden, with a special interest in diseases of the eye. In 1837 he was appointed *Hofrath* (Councillor) and personal physician to the King of Saxony.

students away from the university clinic, and interfered with the proper teaching of the students. By the end of his first year in office Zeis was having to defend himself against gossip, spread by Robert, that impugned his reputation as a surgeon, and shook the confidence of the students in his authority.

On 1 December 1844 he wrote to the pro-rector to lodge a complaint against Robert. On Sunday 24 November he had amputated a leg with multiple fractures and moist gangrene. The next day he demonstrated the amputated limb to those students who had not been at the operation. One of the students asked to take the leg away for further examination. Zeis warned him not to throw away any part of the limb, because this would prejudice the public against dissections. Zeis heard later from Fick (the professor of anatomy, and Zeis' only ally in Marburg) that the student had taken the leg straight to Robert, who had declared that it was not gangrenous, and that it should never have been amputated. Investigation by the pro-rector vindicated Zeis, and Robert was reprimanded for his unacademic conduct. But the gossip continued, and the authorities were led to believe that Zeis, although competent in the theory of surgery, was suspect in the practice. At no other time in his career, however, was there anything but praise for his outstanding skill in operative surgery. He was also involved in disputes with Heusinger over the treatment of surgical patients in the medical clinic. In general, he met nothing but antagonism from his colleagues. His excitable temperament made it impossible for him to compromise, and this contributed to his difficulties, wearing him out, and destroying his peace of mind. In October 1849 he was delighted to receive an invitation to return to Dresden as director of the surgical department of the newly opened City Hospital. He at once sent in his resignation to the Marburg Senate. Robert had offended others on the Faculty, and they refused to recommend him for the chair of surgery. Zeis was succeeded by Wilhelm Roser, who remained in the chair until his death in 1888.

During his eighteen years in Dresden Zeis was respected for his tireless work on behalf of thousands of patients. But his talents were not always appreciated by his contemporaries. He had a quarrelsome nature, with sudden outbursts of temper, and, although these storms quickly subsided, he was often in conflict with his colleagues. As well as his busy surgical practice, he continued and completed his collection of material on plastic surgical operations and their history. He thought that it should be possible to encompass this single branch of surgery, and to provide a definitive catalogue of the scattered literature. He found many errors in the earlier literature, with one author copying from another without checking the original source. He determined to find, and if possible to own, everything that had been written on the subject. This search took much of his time, and he had to expend a great deal of his modest income. He consulted libraries up and down the country, and travelled widely to hunt for difficult items, especially in private collections. He made a complete catalogue of the Royal Library in Dresden, where he found much of his material. His major work on the literature and history of plastic surgery was published in 1863, but there were so many new items that a supplement was needed the following year.[7] Towards the end of his life he took up microscopy, investigating the frequent occurrence of 'blue pus' in his hospital; his last publication was 'On hospital gangrene'. In 1868 he suffered increasing failure of vision, which made him very depressed for fear that he was going blind, and would therefore be unable to work. He died in Dresden on 28 June 1868, collapsing suddenly on his way to the hospital to carry out a hernia operation. He was unmarried.[8]

PLASTIC SURGERY OUTSIDE GERMANY

Zeis was always concerned to defend the rights of Germany and German surgeons against other nations, particularly the French whom he felt had made unjustifiable claims for their part in the development of plastic surgery. If he strafed the French, they certainly gave as good as they got; both parties were criticized for this by the British.[9] It was recognized that major advances were being made in Germany, and that Dieffenbach was the master.[10] But there was no lack of interest in other countries. Zeis, however, found it difficult to see all the English and French journals, and he often had to rely on a review notice in a German journal. This led to omissions in the *Manual*, for which he was

[7] E. Zeis, *Die Literatur und Geschichte der plastischen Chirurgie,* Leipzig (1863); and *Nachträge dazu,* Leipzig (1864) [facsimile, Arnaldo Forni-Editore, Bologna (1963).] The main volume (1863) and its supplement (1864) have been collated and translated, with additions and revisions: T. J. S. Patterson, *The Zeis index and history of plastic surgery*, The McDowell Series of Plastic Surgical Indexes, Vol. 1, Williams and Wilkins, Baltimore (1977).

[8] For a general biography of Zeis see: M. Bille, Nekrolog des Professor Dr. Eduard Zeis, *Sitzungsberichte der Gesellschaft für Natur- und Heilkunde zu Dresden* **2**, 150 (1868–69); T. Gibson, Eduard Zeis (1807–1868) plastic surgeon bibliographer extraordinary, *Br. J. plast. Surg.* **29**, 277 (1976). For details of Zeis' years in Marburg see: K.-F. Kaufmann, *Die ersten 100 Jahre Chirurgie in Marburg,* Diss., Marburg (1963).

[9] *Br. for. med. Rev.* **19**, 398 (1846).

[10] 'the greatest restorer of noses after Tagliacozzi'. *Lancet* **1**, 387 (1834–5).

taken to task by the English and French reviewers.[11] There were also mistakes in citations of foreign articles. Although he was able to correct many of these later,[12] his account of publications and operations outside Germany up to 1838 was incomplete.

In France, Delpech had reconstructed a nose in 1823—the year that three such operations were reported in Europe,[13]—and by 1830 he had carried out 15 reconstructions. His countrymen may have been slow to follow his example—'a singular fact in that land of personal vanity'[14] —but, from 1834, Dieffenbach's visits to Paris and other centres aroused great interest, and encouraged many French surgeons to take up plastic surgery. Phillips, a Belgian, was collecting examples of 'autoplastie' from all over Europe; he described two of Dieffenbach's operations at the Hôpital de la Pitié in Paris in 1834: reconstruction of a scrofulous nose with a flap from the forehead, and reconstruction of the lower eyelid after excision of cancer.[15] Zeis' *Manual* had been preceded by Labat's book on rhinoplasty (1834),[16] and Blandin's *Autoplastie* (1836),[17] although neither of these covered the whole field of plastic surgery.

In England, Hutchison (1818)[18] had carried out the first rhinoplasty after Carpue, and he was followed by Travers (1823), Davies (1824), Liston (1827), Green (1828), Coley and Collis (1831), Syme (1834), Robinson (1835), Fergusson (1835—copying Dieffenbach's method of building up a collapsed nose), Douglas, and Skey (1836). There were a number of review articles and lectures on plastic surgery. Thomson had given the history from Celsus up to the end of the eighteenth century.[19] Lawrence, in his lectures at St. Bartholomew's Hospital in 1829, discussed the history and techniques, and stated that 'some new noses have been made at this hospital in this way'.[20] A review article in

---

[11] 'We would venture to assert that there is scarcely a London or provincial surgeon who has not performed various plastic operations of more or less importance'. On plastic surgery, *Br. for. med. Rev.* **7**, 393 (1839).

[12] See n. 7 above.

[13] Taliacotian operation for a new nose, *Lancet* **4**, 21, 159 (1823–4). The surgeons were Delpech in Montpellier, and John Davies and Benjamin Travers in London.

[14] *Br. for. med. Rev.* **7**, 392 (1839).

[15] C. Phillips, Restoration of the nose and eyelid, *Lancet* **1**, 182 (1834–5); and see p. 137, n. 11.

[16] See p. 16, n. 65. [17] See p. xxvii, n. 33. [18] See p. 52, n. 10.

[19] J. Thomson, *Lectures on inflammation*, Edinburgh, p. 224 (1813).

[20] W. Lawrence, Nature and treatment of injuries, *Lancet* **1**, 521 (1829–30).

1823 gave a full history from the earliest times up to Carpue (1816), and the latest example of rhinoplasty—by Travers (1823).[21] A further article in 1834 was designed to bring up to date those to whom the published works might not be very accessible.[22] However, Spencer Wells, as late as 1854, was lamenting that there was still no major work in English:

it is not a little singular that no work on plastic surgery has yet appeared in the English language. There is too much reason to fear that this want in our literature is connected, either as cause or effect, with a certain inadequate appreciation in this country of what plastic surgery can effect, and some ignorance of what it has effected in Germany, France and Italy.[23]

In Holland, van Onsenoort had reconstructed a nose in 1824; in Italy, Canella (1825) was followed by Signoroni (1833). The news of the Indian operation was published in America in 1806.[24] In 1837 Warren reported the first successful case of a forehead flap,[25] by which time Mütter had already started his work in reconstructive surgery.[26]

Zeis realized that his *Manual* was incomplete. When his later work was published (1863–4), he hoped that this would be the definitive account. But he was afraid that, even after all his efforts, he might still have failed. He comforted himself with the thought that he had collected and sorted the literature as no one had ever done before. In 1838 he noted how much more work was needed to solve many of the surgical problems of the day, but by 1863 he could write that, although new discoveries were still being made:

no-one can doubt that the first half of the nineteenth century will always be recognized in the history of medicine as the Golden Age of plastic surgery, and that future generations will appreciate how hard we have worked to raise the edifice of plastic surgery, so that it may be regarded as complete in all main respects.[27]

Dieffenbach and his contemporaries, with Zeis as Boswell, had worked out the principles of grafting with local skin flaps. Reverdin

---

[21] Nasal operation, *Lancet* **1**, 233 (1823).

[22] *Lancet* **1**, 385 (1834–5).

[23] T. S. Wells, Practical essays on plastic surgery, *Med. Times and Gaz.* **9**, 9 (1854).

[24] Account of the method of supplying artifical noses; as practised by the natives of the Malabar Coast, *Philadelphia Medical Museum* **2**, 343 (1806).

[25] J. M. Warren, Rhinoplastic operation, *Boston med. surg. J.* **16**, 69 (1837).

[26] T. D. Mütter, *Cases of autoplastic,* Philadelphia (1838).

[27] Zeis, *Literatur und Geschichte,* p. viii.

(1869), Ollier (1872), Wolfe (1875), Thiersch (1886), and many others were soon to introduce free skin grafting into clinical practice. The next major advance in the transplantation of skin would be in the First World War, when the correct indications for each type of graft were established.

NOTES ON THIS TRANSLATION

Zeis' book is in two equal parts: the first half contains the general principles of plastic surgery, its history, and indications, and the care of the patient before and after operation; in the second half are the special operative techniques required for the individual parts of the body. The text is long, over-elaborate, and repetitive—'vastly more bulky than is essential for even a full discussion of the various branches of plastic surgery; but this diffuseness is too generally cultivated to be considered a fault in Germany.'[28] Zeis would have answered these criticisms by pointing out that he was writing for surgeons who had no experience of this new specialty. By omitting repetitions and redundancies, and tightening up the text by a greater use of cross-references, I have reduced the total length by about one-third.

Tenotomy was one of Zeis' interests, but even he found it hard to justify its inclusion in a book on plastic surgery; I have shortened this section considerably. I have moved a few shorter passages in other chapters—usually to ensure that the case reports are in the appropriate sections. Zeis put a number of subject-headings within chapters, but these were irregularly scattered; I have added others, particularly to define the case reports, to which he attached great importance. He often used the editors' names as an abbreviated title for a journal, e.g. *Gr. u. W. Jour.* for *Graefe und von Walther's Journal der Chirurgie und Augenheilkunde.* I have altered the titles of journals to conform, as far as possible, to the *World List of Scientific Periodicals.*

By the time that he wrote the *Manual*, Zeis had already collected a large bibliography which was printed at the beginning of the book. He was well aware that this was not complete, particularly for works outside Germany. Some of his citations and some of his historical facts are wrong. He corrected many of these later;[29] I have tried to correct the rest. They occur mostly in the historical sections, but I have added, or amended, a number of references in other chapters. If possible, I have used the English of an original item instead of re-translating Zeis'

---

[28] *Br. for. med. Rev.* **7**, 416 (1839).

[29] See n. 7 above.

German version. I have added biographical notes of some of the more prominent figures, and references to relevant modern authors. My alterations and insertions are in [square brackets].

ACKNOWLEDGEMENTS

Blair Rogers has given me generous support and encouragement to finish this translation in time for the 150th anniversary of the original publication. I would like to thank Charles Webster, Irvine Loudon, and my other colleagues in the Wellcome Unit for the History of Medicine for their good advice at all times. John Waś has translated the Latin quotations from Tagliacozzi, and I would like to thank him and the staff of Oxford University Press for their help.

I am grateful to the Librarian and the photographic department of the Royal College of Surgeons of England for the skill with which the prints for the title and illustrations have been produced from the original copperplates and the stained and faded wood-cuts.

Dr Robert M. Goldwyn and the editorial board of *Plastic and Reconstructive Surgery* have kindly given me permission to quote from pp. xv–xxiv, 1–3, 97, and 105 of T. J. S. Patterson, *The Zeis index and history of plastic surgery*, The Williams and Wilkins Co., Baltimore (1977).

Finally, I would like to remember Frank McDowell, who first drew my attention to the writings of Eduard Zeis, and who did so much to continue Zeis' mission to provide a complete bibliography of plastic surgery.

Oxford T. J. S. P.
1988

PLATES

(Plates fall between pp. 114 and 115 of the text)

FIGURES

Handbuch
der
plastischen Chirurgie

von

Eduard Zeis,

Doctor der Medicin und Chirurgie, praktischem Arzte zu Dresden, Armenarzte, Arzte beim Augenkrankenheilverein, der Kinderheilanstalt, zweitem Arzte der Blindenerziehungsanstalt, der Gesellschaft für Natur- und Heilkunde zu Dresden ordentlichem, und der Hufelandschen med. chir. Gesellschaft zu Berlin correspondirendem Mitgliede.

Nebst

einer Vorrede

von

J. F. Dieffenbach,

Ritter mehrerer Orden,
Doctor der Medicin und Chirurgie, Professor an der Universität und dirigirendem Arzt an der Charité zu Berlin, Mitglied einiger Academien und Gesellschaften.

Mit vielen Holzschnitten und zwei Kupfertafeln.

Berlin.

Gedruckt und verlegt bei G. Reimer.

1838.

ZEIS' MANUAL OF PLASTIC SURGERY

For the ancients would pare the skin, pull it gently together, and fasten it with sutures, and they would attempt nothing more than this. But we make incisions into the skin, separating it from the underlying tissues, so that it is still attached, however, at one point. Then we make a fresh wound by paring the nose, and attach the graft, holding it firmly with sutures. We divide it many days later, carve out nostrils, and complete it with whatever else remains to be done. But lesser surgeons do none of these things.[30]

---

[30] G. Tagliacozzi, *de curtorum chirurgia per insitionem,* Vol. 1, Venice, chapter 10. (1597).
[Gaspare Tagliacozzi (1545–99), was professor of anatomy, surgery (1570–89), and medicine (1590–99) at the university of Bologna. The first edition of *de curtorum*, 2 Vols, (Bindoni) was followed by a pirated edition (Venice, 1597), (Meietti); later editions were Frankfurt (1598), Geneva (1721), and Berlin (1831). There is a facsimile of the Meietti edn by the Libreria Manuel Porrua, Mexico, D. F., Mexico (1972). There has only been one (incomplete) translation into English: A. Read, *Chirurgorum comes; or, The whole practice of chirurgery,* London, (1687)—where the last 21 chapters contain 'the substance of Taliacautius, concerning the supplying of a Nose, Lip, or Ear artificially', translated and added by an unknown author (Read died in 1641). This only covers the second volume—the practical part. There is an abstract of the first volume—the theory—in M. T. Gnudi and J. P. Webster, *The life and times of Gaspare Tagliacozzi*, New York, pp. 197–204 (1950).]

Dedicated to

F. A. von Ammon[31]

and

J. F. Dieffenbach[32]

---

[31] [See n. 6 above.]

[32] [See n. 2 above.]

FOREWORD

Dr Zeis of Dresden has done me the honour of asking me to write a foreword to his work on plastic surgery. I am very happy to do this, but it is superfluous to praise his book, for every reader will soon be convinced of its merits. Dr Zeis has not only collected all that is known of this branch of surgery, but he has added much that is new from his own and von Ammon's experience. I myself have communicated to Dr Zeis relevant material that I have observed and found useful in recent years, in order to support this worthy undertaking.

It is quite unnecessary to say anything here in praise of this branch of surgery, which deals with the reconstruction of deformed parts of the body. Its value has been amply demonstrated in recent times, and it is the brightest bloom in the whole of surgery. By it, surgery has once again been united with physiology, when previously they had been separated by the teachings of the old surgeons, as if by barricades. These have now fallen.

May this work go down to posterity like that of Caspar Taliacotius!

Berlin
28 April 1838 Dieffenbach

AUTHOR'S PREFACE

Some years ago Councillor von Ammon urged me to write a book on plastic surgery, but I thought that it would be too difficult. But when Professor Dieffenbach also requested it, and promised me his support, I set to work. Blandin's book,[33] the first to deal with the whole of plastic surgery, had just appeared. When I reviewed it I found it to be a very superficial work. But I was afraid that I would be pre-empted in Germany, where this book, with its author's delusion that plastic surgery was created by his countrymen, might find a translator as well as supporters. Thus it was necessary to bring out a book quickly, which, while recognizing Carpue's merits,[34] would give Germany the credit for having done most to revive plastic surgery. It would show the position that this branch of surgery has now reached, and serve as a primer for the inexperienced surgeon. But it would also be useful to the experienced surgeon, and save him the trouble of collecting all the very scattered source material.

I have found it very difficult to define the boundaries of plastic surgery, and I have been criticized for this. For example, I have omitted operations to join abnormally divided parts, such as hare-lip and cleft palate, because no new tissue is introduced. The cure of a torn perineum, and the closure of wounds of the gut, which the French dignify with the name 'enteroplasty', must also be omitted, much as I would like to have included Dieffenbach's successful joining of the two ends after excision of a large piece of intestine. It may seem a contradiction to include fistulae of the trachea, male urethra, and bladder, and the closure of hernial openings. I can only justify this in that I have been concerned more with the technique of the operation than with its purpose, and that the operations described here are all carried out by

---

33 P. F. Blandin, *Autoplastie, ou restauration des parties du corps, qui ont été détruites, à la faveur d'un emprunt fait à d'autres parties plus ou moins éloignées*, Paris (1836). [Philippe-Frédéric Blandin (1798–1849), anatomist, and professor of operative surgery, Hôtel Dieu, Paris.]

34 J. C. Carpue, *An account of two successful operations for restoring a lost nose from the integuments of the forehead in the cases of two officers of His Majesty's Army*, London (1816). [Joseph Constantine Carpue (1764–1846), surgeon of the York Hospital, Chelsea, the National Vaccine Institution, and St. Pancras Infirmary. See biography in: *Lancet* **1**, 166 (1846).]

transplantation, and are thus part of plastic surgery. Stomatoplasty[35] is included, but not the opening-up of other abnormal fusions, as of the anus or vagina. I have, however, discussed tenotomy, although strictly speaking this is not plastic surgery, for the formation of new tissue between the cut ends of a tendon is the work of nature and not, as in transplantation, of art. But I feel that I have done the reader a service by giving him the up-to-date treatment in a subject that is on the boundary between surgery and orthopaedics.

I know that many surgeons, who have no experience of plastic operations, are not yet convinced of their value. My intention is to give a true picture of what plastic surgery can do, without exaggerating or raising expectations which it cannot fulfil. Only he who is himself convinced can convince others, and I hope to persuade many surgeons, who up to now have had little faith in plastic surgery, to give it a trial.

I hope that I will not be criticized for including case histories, but an actual case often attracts more attention than the abstract description of the technique of an operation. I am indebted to my publisher for allowing me as many illustrations as I wished. I have tried not to abuse this, so as not to increase the price of the book. I chose woodcuts because it is easier to compare the figure with the text when they are near each other, rather than pulling out folded copperplates. People are often too lazy to do this, so that they then fail to understand the passage properly. There are only a few lines in each illustration, for it is not my intention to give portraits of individual patients, but simply to represent the technique of the operation. There are two copperplates [between pages 114 and 115], which will, I hope, help those who have never seen a transplantation.

Councillor von Ammon and Professor Dieffenbach have given me much good advice in the preparation of this book. The former has allowed me the full use of his library, and the latter has given me verbal and written information on his latest, as yet unpublished, operations, which are soon to appear in the fifth volume of his *chirurgische Erfahrungen*.[36]

Dresden
April 1838 The author

[35] [Opening-up a mouth closed by scarring.]

[36] [This volume was never published. Dieffenbach also failed to send Zeis the material that he had promised, but inserted the appropriate pages in Zeis' book during its publication in Berlin, without showing them to him beforehand. Dieffenbach set out his work on plastic surgery at length in his: *Die operative Chirurgie,* Vol. 1, Leipzig, (1845). This was reviewed in detail by Spencer Wells in: *Br. for. med. Rev.* **21**, 285 (1846).]

I

INTRODUCTION

DEFINITION

Plastic surgery is the branch of operative surgery that deals with the restoration, with living tissue, of parts that have been destroyed. This is only possible to a limited extent, depending upon the size and complexity of the part. Arms and legs cannot be reconstructed, and there are various artificial aids to improve their function and appearance. Some cripples use these with advantage, but others regard them as instruments of torture, and the majority cannot afford them. This is not part of plastic surgery, and it will not be discussed in this book. But operative surgery can replace missing noses, lips, cheeks, eyelids, and various other parts, by transplantation of skin, so that the appearance is improved, and the function is more-or-less restored. Plastic surgery can still only repair a defect with skin, so that the reconstruction will only partly resemble the original, particularly if it contained other tissues—cartilage, bone, muscle, mucous membrane, hair, etc. For this art can never restore the perfection that Nature has created.

Regeneration is more complete in the lower animals than in the higher, and it is the same for the tissues—the more highly developed, the less the power of regeneration. In man, even though a hair or a nail will re-grow if its root is undamaged, a bony defect is only replaced by callus, and a skin defect by scar, which are of a much lower order than true bone and skin; wounds of muscle can only heal by fibrous tissue. Even this does not occur in the more highly developed organs, and there is no trace of regeneration in an eye, a tooth, a finger-tip, or the tip of the nose, as there would be in a crab that had lost a claw. Plastic surgery uses the inherent power of the organism to heal, either by first intention or by suppuration and granulation, and relies on Nature to keep a flap of skin alive on a small pedicle until it has completely healed into its new site. Medicine can achieve nothing without the help of Nature; 'this is the function of art: to obey Nature if she is acting correctly, and to constrain and correct her, if she is deviating from her true path'.[1] The plastic surgeon raises a flap of skin to a certain point,

[1] Tagliacozzi, *de curtorum,* Vol. 2, Chapter 19, p. 69.

beyond which he must not go, sutures it into close contact with a raw surface, and the power of healing does the rest. But he will get better results if the operation has been carefully planned and carried out, and if he understands the physiological and pathological conditions after an operation, and how to manage them.

Plastic operations are, in general, characterized by transplantation of skin, but there are also some where the skin is simply advanced or folded over. The separation of conjoined parts, or parts drawn together by scarring, may also be included, e.g. enlarging the contracted mouth by re-lining the lips. But operations for conditions such as anal atresia are not plastic surgery. In many cases it is difficult to draw the line. But this has not prevented me from including some operations that are not obviously plastic, such as the reunion of completely separated parts and the closure of various fistulae, and omitting others. Hare-lip and the repair of the soft palate are at least as closely related to plastic surgery as episiorrhaphy,[2] but they have been fully described by other authors. This may seem illogical, but it is a matter of personal judgement of what to select.

JUSTIFICATION OF THE NAME 'PLASTIC SURGERY'

I have chosen 'plastic surgery' as the most appropriate name for this subject. Tagliacozzi, and many after him, used *chirurgia curtorum (per insitionem)* and *chirurgia decoratoria*. Recently the terms 'blepharoplasty', 'cheiloplasty', etc. have been coined, following the style of 'rhinoplasty'.[3] But it is wrong to use 'urethroplasty' and 'cystoplasty' for the transplantation of skin to close vesical, urethral, or vesico-vaginal fistulae, as these terms imply more than this. As a general term, 'organoplasty' has been suggested, but the imperfect relation of a reconstructed part to the original has already been discussed.

> For it is clear how far the limits of Art extend, and how great is the majesty of Nature, how hard it is to approach her, and how far superior she is to Art. It is impossible, however diligently you study the tissues, to attain to the secret and inimitable character of Nature. For this reason, anyone who wishes will easily find much to criticize in this operation.[4]

It cannot be claimed that an organ has been created when rhinoplasty or blepharoplasty has been carried out, and 'organoplasty' is

---

[2] [Suturing the labia to control prolapse of the uterus.]

[3] [*'Rhinoplastik'*—first used by von Gräfe (1818).]

[4] Tagliacozzi, *de curtorum*, Vol. 1, Chapter 24, p. 69.

even more pretentious. Von Ammon suggested 'morioplasty',[5] but *morion* (a piece of the body) is even vaguer than *organon*. The terms used by the French—*'transplantation'*, *'ente animale'*, *'greffe animale'*, and *'anaplastie'*—are equally unsuitable, as they only describe one type of plastic operation; some plastic operations are carried out without any transplantation. But the worst of all is *'autoplastie'*, used by Blandin for operations where the skin is taken from the same individual, as distinct from those where the skin is taken from another individual, which he calls *'heteroplastie'*. This distinction is unnecessary in a general term for plastic operations, since this second type of grafting (which is said to be used in India, although even there it appears to be the less common method) was only done very rarely in Europe, and was then the subject of many fabulous accounts, at a time when people were very much taken up with magic. If it were a practicable method, it should be discussed in any comprehensive book on plastic surgery. But the term is quite wrongly chosen. Anyone hearing it for the first time would not know that Blandin was referring to taking skin from the same individual for reconstruction. It sounds more like spontaneous generation.

I have not insisted on a one-word name, and I have chosen 'plastic surgery' because it is comprehensive and easy to understand.

THE RELATION OF PLASTIC SURGERY TO MEDICINE AND TO THE REST OF SURGERY

The recent struggle to bring medicine and surgery closer together has already had beneficial results. While they were once thought to be opposed, they now work more closely together. The physician, even if he never does major operations himself, can no longer scorn surgery, as something that he does not need to know about, if he is to avoid the charge of ignorance, even among laymen. The best surgeons, at least in Germany, have earned the respect of the physicians, partly by their personal qualities, and partly by the way surgery is now practised, so that surgery is no longer subordinate to medicine, but equal to it. Only in outdated institutions, which should be changed by legislation, is minor surgery still being done by barber-surgeons (who, with their shoddy techniques, should have nothing to do with it), instead of by surgeons of the Second Class. But the special quality that turns a doctor into a surgeon is inborn, and this will always prevent closer fusion of surgery and medicine. This is no bad thing—when there are too many

[5] F. A. von Ammon, Beiträge zur Morioplastik, *Magazin ges. Heilk.* **32,** 162 (1830).

surgeons, there are not enough operations to go round. No one can get the necessary experience, nor keep his hand in, so that no one becomes expert.

A doctor, even if he has no inclination towards a particular specialty, may find that one or more successful cases will attract other similar patients to him, and soon he will unwittingly have become an ear specialist or a good pox doctor. The patients themselves realize the great store of knowledge that is needed to become equally competent in all branches of medicine, and they have more faith in someone whom they know to be a specialist. Many a young doctor starting in practice may have felt strongly inclined towards surgery or ophthalmology, but, because of the plate on his door, he cannot get the sort of patients that he would like. It seems that ophthalmology, although closely related to surgery, will always be a separate specialty. Obstetrics is too tiring and time-consuming for every doctor, and orthopaedic patients will always make their way to those who happily busy themselves with trusses and splints. It is the same with internal medicine—some doctors excel in the treatment of lung, heart, or nervous diseases, and such specialization, if not carried too far, has led to many of medicine's greatest discoveries. Few doctors can be competent in all branches of medicine, and it is better that they should specialize in one, rather than cover all superficially. It is natural that, in surgery, which needs such varied manual skills, there is this tendency to specialize. Cutting for stone was once practised by a separate class of surgeons: the Marianis, Colots, Franco,[6] Frère Côme, Rau, and their followers. At the present time, Civiale, Amussat, Heurteloup, and others in Paris are concerned mainly, but not exclusively, with lithotrity. It was the same with many other operations, and with *chirurgia curtorum* several centuries ago, which remained in the hands of the Brancas and Bojanis, who kept it secret. Tagliacozzi wished to make it more widely known, but he did not achieve this in his time.

Plastic surgery has recently been taken up by our leading surgeons, and has made such rapid strides that it can never sink back into its former oblivion. But many surgeons have still not accepted it. This book, with its account of what has been achieved up to now, is not intended to turn all surgeons into plastic surgeons. Its chief purpose is to increase the number of plastic surgeons, and to make the subject

[6] [Pierre Franco, originator of the high lithotomy, was also noted for his reconstruction of a large defect of the cheek: *Traité des hernies contenant une ample déclaration de toutes leurs espèces et autres excellentes parties de la chirurgie,* Lyons, p. 462 (1561).

more widely known, for the literature is so scattered that anyone who is interested might not be able to lay his hands on it all.

2

THE HISTORY OF PLASTIC SURGERY

THE EARLIEST TIMES

The first traces of plastic surgery are to be found in India, where cutting off the nose was a common punishment for stealing. All this is lost in the mists of antiquity, and we only have the very dubious information that the caste of Koomas, a sort of lower priest, descended from the Brahmins, and who still possess the art of reconstructing noses, lips, and ears, have practised this from the earliest times.[1] Graham tells us that:

> the profession of astrology, and the task of making almanacks, belong to degraded Brahmins, and the occupations of teaching military exercises and physic, as well as the trades of potters, weavers, braziers, fishermen and workers in shells belong also to the descendants of Brahmins.[2]

It is not surprising that plastic surgery is in the hands of the Koomas, for astrology and medicine are closely related in India, as indeed all over the East.

It is difficult to find out if rhinoplasty spread from India to the rest of Asia, and whether the Egyptians, Greeks, and Romans knew how to reconstruct missing parts. Galen said that the priests in Egypt made noses, but kept the technique secret. The operation for hare-lip and the closure of clefts in the lips and ears that he mentions cannot really be counted as plastic operations.[3] Celsus' operation was also not carried out by transplantation, for he only advanced local skin to close wide clefts in the upper lip:

> the defect is converted into a square; from the inner angles of this, transverse incisions are made so that the part on one side of the square is completely separated from that on the opposite side.

---

[1] [Koomars are potters and tile-makers. The Artist of Poona was a member of this caste—see n. 40 below.]

[2] M. Graham [later Lady Calcott], *Letters on India*, London, p. 278 (1814).

[3] C. Galen, *Methodus medendi*, Book 14, Chapter 16, editio Kühniana, Leipzig, (1827).

I can explain this famous passage with the help of Fig. 1: after excising the edges of the cleft, horizontal incisions (*b* and *c*) are made from the angle (*a*) through the full thickness of the lip. This gives a flap on each side. Celsus continues:

now the tissues which have been freed are brought together. If this is not possible, two additional semilunar incisions should be made, at some distance from the original incisions and concave towards them, but only dividing the skin. These enable the parts to be more easily brought together.[4]

These curved relieving incisions are shown as *d–d*. When these incisions are necessary, the operation comes nearer to plastic surgery, as it produces new tissue by lateral shifting, and is not simply the closure of a cleft.[5] But this is the only trace of plastic surgery to be found in Europe in olden times.

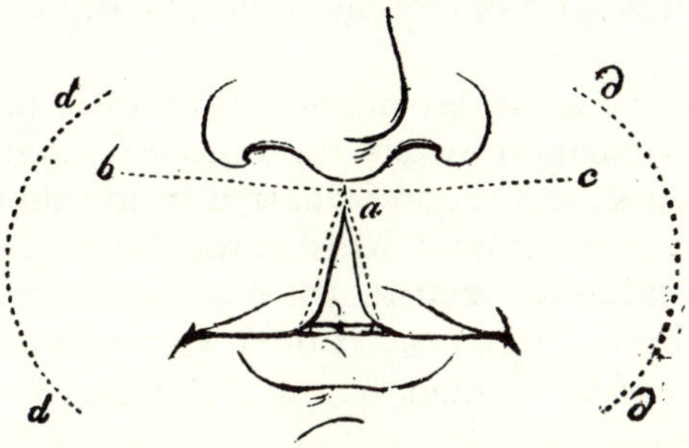

Fig 1

There was then a long interval. Paulus Aegineta only described freeing and advancing skin for the treatment of deformities of the ears and lips:

mutilations of the ears and lips, called by the Greeks 'colobomata', are cured in this way. First the skin is freed on the under side, then the edges of the wound are drawn together, and the calloused part is removed. Then the stitches holding them into place have to be applied.[6]

PLASTIC SURGERY IN ITALY, TAGLIACOZZI

At the end of the fourteenth, or beginning of the fifteenth, century Branca, a surgeon in Sicily, knew how to replace noses, lips, and ears, as reported by Ranzano.[7] A contemporary of Branca, the poet Elisio Calenzio in Naples, wrote about him to a friend:

---

4 A. C. Celsus, curta in auribus, labrisque ac naribus, quomodo sarciri et curari possint, *de medicina* Book 7, Chapter 9.

5 [Zeis claimed that he was the first to give a surgically intelligible translation of this passage. He later expanded this in *Drei chirurgische Abhandlungen über die plastische Chirurgie des Celsus*, Dresden and Leipzig (1843).]

6 Paul of Aegina [middle of the seventh century AD], curta in auribus et labiis quomodo sarciri possint, *opera*, Leyden, Book 6. Chapter 26, p. 583 (1589). [F. Adams, *The seven books of Paulus Aegineta*, for the Sydenham Society, London, (1854).]

7 P. Ranzano (1420–92), Bishop of Lucera in Capitania, wrote *Annales mundi*, which are preserved in manuscript in the library of the Dominicans in Palermo. His account of the Brancas is given in the eighth book of his history of the world, and in Vincenzio Auria, *La Sicilia inventrice con li divertimenti geniali di Dr Mongitore*, Palermo, Book 6. Chapter 3. p. 10 (1704).

Orpianus, if you want your nose restored, come here to me. For sure, men think it is a miracle. The Sicilian, Brancha, a man of outstanding genius, has learnt how to ingraft a nose, which he either replaces from the arm, or he fixes on one borrowed from a servant. When I saw this I decided to write to you, thinking that no news could be more welcome. If you come, rest assured that you will return home with as splendid a nose as you desire.[8]

It is not known where Branca learned this art, and whether he knew about the Indian technique of rhinoplasty, or whether he discovered it himself; he kept his technique a secret, and there is no further information about it.[9] His son, Antonius, and one of his pupils, Balthasar Pavono, also practised the art.[10]

Next came the Bojani family,[11] Vincent, his nephew Bernard, and Bernard's son Peter, in Tropaea, a Neapolitan city.[12] But none of them left a description of their operations, and the information from other authors is very incomplete, and even incorrect.[13] Most of them thought that the muscle of the arm was used to reconstruct the nose—an error still made even today in cities where rhinoplasty is often carried out, and one that is more readily believed by laymen than that skin alone is all that is needed to replace a nose.

Among the writers of those times who mention rhinoplasty are Benedetti.[14] Gourmelenus,[15] and Vesalius.[16] Ambroise Paré doubted that completely separated parts could be united, but spoke of a surgeon in Italy who reconstructed noses from the muscle of the arm.[17] There is

---

[8] S. Gourmelenus, *Chirurgicae artis* Vol. 1, Paris, p. 72 (1580).

[9] [Zeis later found a more detailed contemporary account of the Brancas, father and son, by Bartolomeo Fazio (d. 1457), *De viris illustribus liber,* Florence (1745).]

[10] V. Coronelli, *Bibliotheca universale,* Vol. 6, Venice p. 1034 (1706).

[11] [Sometimes called Vianeo.]

[12] N. F. J. Eloy, *Dictionnaire historique de médecine ancienne et moderne,* Vol. 4, Mons, p. 358 (1778).

[13] [Zeis later concluded, from other contemporary accounts, e.g. G. Barri, *De antiquitate et situ Calabriae,* Franfurt (1600), that the Bojanis were still practising rhinoplasty at the time that Tagliacozzi had completed his first four cases.]

[14] A. Benedetti. *Anatomia sive historia corporis humani,* Book 6, Venice, Chapter 39, p. 51 (1502). [Benedetti's instructions were quoted by Tagliacozzi, *de curtorum,* Vol. 1, Chapter 19. p. 62.]

[15] See n. 8 above.

[16] A. Vesalius, *Chirurgiae magnae,* Vol. 3, Leyden, Chapter 9, p. 982 (1725). [Vesalius was one of those who stated that muscle was used for the reconstruction, but this error may have been fault of the editor of the Venice (1568) edition (see Gnudi and Webster, p. 122).]

[17] A. Paré, *Opera chirurgica,* Book 22, Frankfurt, Chapter 2. p. 650 (1594). [First edition, Paris (1582). See also M. N. Saad and J. N. Barron, Ambroise Paré. His contributions to plastic surgery, *Plastic reconstr. Surg.* **46,** 271 (1970).]

nothing to suggest that any of these surgeons carried out plastic operations, and the art would have disappeared again if it had not been for Tagliacozzi, who, unselfishly, without trying to keep his work secret, and inspired only by the wish to help unhappy, deformed patients, studied rhinoplasty in a truly scientific manner, handing this down in his writings:

> for we are not the sort to wish our art to remain with us, as if enchained, but rather we wish it to extend even to foreign nations, for which reason we have given everyone the opportunity to watch while we are operating.[18]

Gaspare Tagliacozzi, born in Bologna in 1545, was professor of anatomy and medicine there. He practised rhinoplasty over a long period, and was widely renowned as a restorer of noses before he published *de chirurgia curtorum per insitionem* in Venice in 1597. He was always concerned to spread the word about rhinoplasty, and to instruct other surgeons. He thought that he was the first to take the skin from a distant part of the body. But we now know that Branca also took the skin from the arm, so that Tagliacozzi was wrong about this. After his death, in 1599, the City Council of Bologna honoured his memory by a statue, holding a nose in its hand, which is still in the anatomical theatre in Bologna. He is less well-known as an anatomist, although his contemporaries also respected him for this.[19] There have always been people who have criticized him, finding his book tedious and confusing, and regarding him as boastful, because thirteen laudatory poems are printed in the front of his book. One has only to examine the book to be convinced that he had a knowledge of basic physiology, and that he wrote with good taste and enthusiasm, and to realize that he was only conforming to the custom of his day by having several unnecessary quotations, and the laudatory poems from his friends, included in his book.

THE DECLINE OF PLASTIC SURGERY AFTER TAGLIACOZZI

But there were only a few who copied him. One of his pupils, Cortesi, professor of surgery at Messina, described Tagliacozzi's and his own,

---

[18] Letter from Tagliacozzi to Mercuriale, 22 February 1586, in H. Mercuriale, *de decoratione,* Frankfurt, p. 116 (1587). [Tagliacozzi stresses that skin only, and not muscle, is used for the reconstruction. He names four patients for whom he has made noses, and who all prefer their new noses to the natural ones.]

[19] J. Schenk von Grafenberg, *Observationum medicarum,* Vol. 1, Frankfurt, p. 200 (1609). [See also p. xxii, n. 30.]

modified, technique.[20] Fabry von Hilden reported that Griffon, a surgeon in Lausanne, had reconstructed the nose of a beautiful virgin, who, in 1590, had fallen into the hands of some rough soldiers who would have ravished her; to frustrate them she cut off her nose[21] (certainly a good way of putting off an importunate lover). Two years later, before Tagliacozzi's work was published, Griffon, who had learned the art from a travelling Italian, made her a nose from the skin of her arm, which was so successful that it was hard to tell it from the normal. The girl, unmarried, was still living in Lausanne in 1613. Her nose was in good condition, and it only went a little livid in very cold weather. Fabry von Hilden mentions another rhinoplasty by Griffon, on a girl who was married in 1602, so that it is clear that this is a different case from the first.[22] Thomas Feyens came from Antwerp to Bologna in 1590, and learned Tagliacozzi's technique, which he included in his book.[23] Molinetti stated that his father had restored the nose of a Polish nobleman in Venice in 1625.[24] There are no other attempts at reconstructive operations to be found, and Griffon's two cases seem to be the only ones to have been treated outside Italy.

There followed another long interval when nothing was happening in plastic surgery. Rhinoplasty was regarded as a painful and dangerous operation, and condemned as unnecessary. It was thought to be more convenient, and just as satisfactory, to wear a nose made of silver or wood, and no-one dared to follow Tagliacozzi's example. The whole subject soon became embellished with fables. Tagliacozzi had stated that it was impracticable to make a nose from the skin of another person, and he always used only the patient's own skin. It is not known whether other surgeons at that time took skin from other people. Tagliacozzi described the difficulty of keeping two people so close to each other until union had occurred. In spite of this, there were stories of noses that had fallen off when the previous owner of the piece of skin died. Van Helmont's account was widely believed: a man of Brussels had a nose made by Tagliacozzi from the arm of a porter; after thirteen months he noticed that his nose felt cold, and a few days later it became gangrenous. Enquiries were made, and it was found that the porter had died at the same time. Van Helmont referred to eye-witnesses who

---

[20] G. B. Cortesi, *Miscellaneorum medicinalium decades denae,* Vol. 3, Messina, p. 80 (1625).

[21] W. Fabry von Hilden, *Opera quae exstant omnia,* Frankfurt, p. 214 (1646).

[22] Ibid. p. 1006.

[23] T, Feyens, *de praecipuis artis chirurgicae controversiis.* Frankfurt, p. 99 (1649).

[24] 24 A. Molinetti, *Dissertationes anatomico-pathologicae,* Vol. 4, Venice, p. 174 (1675).

would vouch for it.[25] It is true that harmful influences, such as cold, could cause a reconstructed nose to die after a long time, but there are no recent examples of this.

Fludd has further embroidered this story,[26] but nowadays no-one believes in such a connection between a piece of transplanted skin and its former owner. In the same vein, but more light-hearted, is the passage in *Hudibras*:

So learned *Talicotius* from
The brawny Part of Porter's Bum
Cut Supplemental Noses, which
Would last as long as Parent Breech:
But when the Date of *Nock* was out,
Off dropt the Sympathetick Snout.[27]

Best of all was Bickersteth [sic], who gave a fanciful account of Tagliacozzi's operations, and used this as a warning to the young bloods of London of the dangers of syphilis.[28] Blegny told of a man, whose nose had been lopped off several days before, who had the freshly cut-off nose of his servant attached in its place, and that this fell off when the servant died. Blegny himself doubted the truth of this tale.[29] Jessen's account of rhinoplasty does not indicate that he practised this himself.[30] But it is surprising that he gives an exact description of the operation for reconstruction of the foreskin, which is nowhere else to be found, so that it seems to be his own discovery.[31]

At the beginning of the eighteenth century people cast doubt on even the most trustworthy accounts of the reunion of completely separated parts of the body, and there were many surgeons who regarded Tagliacozzi's art as pure fable. There was certainly no lack of opportunity to put it to the test, but no-one had the courage. Reneaume [de la Garanne] proposed that the length of the Taliacotian method should be reduced by combining the two operations on the arm, which Tagliacozzi separated by 14 days, but he never carried this out himself.[32]

[25] J. B. van Helmont, *Opera omnia*, Frankfurt, p. 707 (1682).

[26] R. Fludd, *Defense of weapon-salve or the squeezing of Parson Foster's Spunge*, (London, p. 132 (1635).

[27] [S. Butler, *Hudibras*, (London, p. 10 (1710) (*Nock* = backside.) Zeis printed the German translation by D. W. Soltau, (Königsberg, 1797). There is also a translation by Voltaire.]

[28] The lucubrations of Isaac Bickerstaff Esq., *The Tatler*, **4**, 313 (1710).]

[29] N. de Blegny, *Zodiacus medico-gallicus*, Geneva, p. 75 (1682).

[30] J. von Jessen, *Institutiones chirurgicae*, Wittenberg, p. 100 (1601).

[31] See p. 182, n. 3.

[32] R. de la Garanne, Sur la réparation de quelques parties du corps humain mutilées, *Hist. Acad. r. Sci.* **4**, 32 (Paris, 1721).

Dionis,[33] and Heister,[34] were among the principal doubters of the possibility of reunion of separated parts, or the repair of missing parts with skin. In 1742, the Medical Faculty in Paris debated the thesis: *an curtae nares ex brachio reficiendae?*[35] The proponent answered in the affirmative, but the Faculty declared that Tagliacozzi's doctrine was a fabrication, and that a transplanted piece of skin must die when its former owner died.[36]

THE INDIAN OPERATION

This was the position at the end of the eighteenth century, when reports of the reconstruction of noses in India reached Europe. A pariah, called Cowasjee, a bullock-driver with the English army, had been taken prisoner with four soldiers in 1792 by Sultan Tippoo, who had punished them by cutting off their noses and hands, and sending them back to the Bombay Army as a warning to traitors. Leaves had been put on the stumps of their arms to stop the bleeding, but there was nothing on their noses. In this pitiful state they reached Poona, where their wounds were healed. Some time later a native merchant, selling oil-cloth, came to the house of the British Resident, Sir Charles Malet. The merchant had had his nose reconstructed after it had been cut off, as he admitted, by the executioner for adultery. Sir Charles Malet sent for the surgeon, who lived four hundred miles away; he was thought to be the only restorer of noses in India, and this art was hereditary in his family. Two surgeons from Bombay, Thomas Cruso and James Findlay, with Colonel Ward,[37] witnessed the operation.[38]

A pattern of the nose was made in wax, laid on the forehead, and a line drawn round it. The surgeon then dissected up this flap, leaving it attached only between the eyebrows. The stump of the nose was freshened, and an incision was made in the upper lip. The flap was

---

33 P. Dionis, *Cours d'opérations de chirurgie,* (Brussels, p. 403 (1708).

34 L. Heister, *Institutiones chirurgicae,* Vol. 2 (Amsterdam, p. 623 (1750).

35 [Whether mutilated noses can be restored from the arm?]

36 P.-F. Percy, *Dictionaire des sciences médicales,* Vol. 12, Paris, p. 343 (1815).

37 [But 'there seems to be no basis for believing that an official prohibition of plastic procedures was ever made by the Faculty of Medicine at Paris' (Gnudi and Webster, p, 307).]

37 [Cruso and Findlay were surgeons in the East India Company's Bombay Army; Ward was Cowasjee's commanding officer at the time he was captured.]

38 *The Hircarrah or Madras Gazette,* 5 August 1794.

turned half round on its pedicle, and laid with its edge in the incision on the nose. No sutures were used, and the flap was only held in place with dressings of *terra japonica* softened with water and spread on five or six slips of cloth. For the first four days no other dressing was used, but this was then replaced by cloth dipped in *ghee* (a kind of butter). The patient had to lie on his back for five or six days. On the tenth day pledgets of soft cloth were put into the nostrils to keep them open, and on the twenty-fifth day the pedicle was divided. The account of this case has an illustration of Cowasjee before and after the operation.[39]

Pennant also mentioned this case, and stated that the nose made by the 'Artist of Poona' was so secure that the patient could sneeze and blow it without the danger of it falling off.[40] Carpue learned from Dr.Barry, who had been a long time in the East Indies, that the operation, which he had witnessed, lasted one-and-a-half hours. The surgeon used an old razor, which, 'being continually blunted in dissection, was every moment re-set'. Tow was used to support the nose, but there was no columella to separate the nostrils. The English surgeon, Lucas, who learned the technique from the Indians, carried it out several times successfully in India, as reported by Major Heitland.[41]

In 1814 Carpue succeeded in finding a suitable case for rhinoplasty, which he had long wished to carry out, and which he had been recommending to his students for fifteen years. He restored an officer's nose which had been destroyed by the misuse of mercury.[42] Soon afterwards a second case presented: an officer who, among multiple wounds received at the battle of Albuera in 1810, had lost his nose and part of his cheek,[43] Carpue's account of these two cases was soon translated into German.[44]

In 1817, Reiner, in Munich, reconstructed a nose by the Indian method. When Sprengel saw the new nose on the tenth day after the operation it was soundly healed, still red but not flat, with a well-shaped columella and nostrils; the pedicle was not very prominent, and the defect in the forehead had already shrunk.[45]

---

39 *Gentleman's Magazine* **64,** p. 891 (1.794). [The next issue (December, p. 1093) contained a letter pointing out that the Taliacotian operation was not unknown in Europe, The news of the Indian operation reached America in 1806—see p. xiv, n. 24.]

40 T. Pennant, *The View of Hindoostan,* Vol. 2, London, p. 237 (1798).

41 Carpue, *Two successful operations,* p.40.

42 See p. 47.

43 See p. 49.

44 H. S, Michaelis, *Geschiche t zweier gelungenen Fälle. wo der Verlust der Nase vermittelst der Stirnhaut ersetzt wurde,* Berlin, (1817) [with a foreword by von Gräfe].

45 K. Sprengel, *Geschichte der Chirurgie,* Vol. 2, Halle, 1819), p. 218.

A second method of reconstruction of the nose, which is said to be common in India, is to transplant a completely separated piece of skin to the face. After the stump of the nose has been prepared, an area on the buttock is beaten with a wooden slipper until it is quite swollen. This increases the vital power of the piece of skin, which is detached with its subcutaneous tissue, and fastened to the face with sticking-plaster.[46] It is surprising that Carpue, who made the most detailed investigation of rhinoplasty in India, did not mention this method.[47] But even more because there had been so much talk in Europe about Tagliacozzi and his contemporaries using the skin from the backside of another person to replace a missing part. Whether this method of reconstruction is really used in India or not, its feasibility has been demonstrated by Bünger,[48] and the climate in India should be much more favourable to the successful reunion of completely separated parts than it is over here.

GRÄFE AND THE ITALIAN OPERATION

Almost at the same time as Carpue, and before he had learned of his work, Grafe,[49] in 1816, used the Italian method to reconstruct the nose of a soldier, lost by a sabre-cut at Montmartre.[50] In 1811 he had made a new nose-tip for a girl from the adjacent parts of the face.[51] In his subsequent cases he modified Tagliacozzi's technique by combining the division of the flap and the attachment to the nose into one stage, calling this the 'German' method.[52]

PLASTIC SURGERY IN EUROPE UP TO 1838

In this way rhinoplasty, and with it plastic surgery in general, was created for the second time, never again to be forgotten. It is now being

---

[46] [Blandin, *Autoplastie,* p. 14 gives H. Dutrochet's account of this operation, as witnessed by his brother-in-law, who was in command of the army of an Indian prince. This was first published in *Gaz. Santé, Paris,* no. 9) (1817).]

[47] Gräfe mentions it in his foreword to Michaelis' translation of Carpue [see n. 44 above].

[48] See p. 21, n. 20.

[49] [Carl Ferdinand von Gräfe (1787-1840)—first professor and director of surgery in Berlin (1810), and Director-General of the Army Medical Services. With von Walther he founded (1820) the *Journal der Chirurgie und Augenheilkunde,* See also: Memoir of Baron Graefe, *Lancet,* **1,** 969 (1833-34); and B. O. Rogers, Carl Ferdinand von Graefe (1787-1840), *Plastic. reconstr, Surg.* **46,** 554 (1970).]

[50] C. F. von Gräfe, *Rhinoplastik, oder die Kunst den Verlust der Nase organisch zu ersetzen,* Berlin, p. 174 (1818).

[51] Ibid. p. 22.

[52] See p. 38.

perfected by the many famous surgeons who have taken it up, to the relief of the endless sufferings of mankind. For even if the rest of surgery can show operations, such as the repair of hernias, excision of tumours, ligature of major arteries, and many others, which restore the patient to full health, yet in other cases, even after the most beneficial and curative operations, such as amputation, castration, and trepanning, the patient is left deformed. But this surgery is life-saving, and happy the man who knows how to restore his brethren to life and health.[53] Plastic surgery is hardly ever indicated for such life-threatening diseases. But this does not make it inferior to the rest of surgery. It may not save lives, but it restores happiness, leaving its patients in a more perfect state than before, by reconstructing individual parts, and restoring normal function. After a rhinoplasty the patient can smell again, and sometimes even hearing is improved. He can blow his nose like anybody else, and, most important of all, he no longer has to hide himself away from people who would run at the sight of him. When his treatment is finished he leaves the surgeon with joy and gratitude for the courage and strenuous efforts which have restored him to the company of his fellows.[54]

Only lack of experience of what plastic surgery can do, still makes many surgeons condemn this branch of surgery. Patients who could be helped are neglected because there is no surgeon nearby who is prepared to undertake plastic operations. But it is to be hoped that the time is not far distant when a surgeon will be ashamed to admit that he cannot carry out plastic operations as skilfully as any others.[55]

Germany will not allow herself to be robbed of the fame of having done the most for plastic surgery since its revival. It is surprising that Carpue's shining example has not been followed up better in England.[56] Apart from a rhinoplasty by Hutchison in 1818,[57] and

[53] 'For of greater importance are those things that are essential, while after these come those that are useful, and then those that are beautiful.' Tagliacozzi, *de curtorum*, 2. Chapter 16. p. 59.

[54] 'What could be more admirable than to exert oneself to shape tissues and form features, to restore to its former function a part that has been destroyed?' ibid. Book 2, Chapter 16, p. 57.

[55] 'Men often abhor something because it is new, unless it comes from Troy, but this is a stupid way to think,' ibid. Book 2, Chapter 13. p. 45.

[56] [Carpue was distinguished as a teacher of anatomy; he wrote on anatomy, the high operation for stone, and medical electricity, but nothing on plastic surgery after 1816.]

[57] See p. 52, n. 10.

reconstruction of the nose and upper lip by Davies in 1823,[58] there seems to have been nothing more,[59] except Syme's closure of a hole in the nose.[60]

In Germany, however, Gräfe's example has been followed by von Ammon, Beck, Benedict, Bünger, Chelius, Dzondi, Fricke, Heidenreich, Reiner, Ruppius, Rust, Textor, von Walther, Werneck, and myself. But above all others, Dieffenbach has devised a host of new and brilliantly thought-out operations for deformities of all sorts, which are giving highly successful results, and raising expectations of even further advances in the art.[61]

In France, Delpech[62] introduced plastic surgery in 1818 with a huge oscheoplasty,[63] and later with reconstructions of the lip and nose, at first by the Italian, and later by the Indian, method.[64] According to Labat,[65] Mouleau in Marseilles, and Thomain in Aix were the next to carry out plastic operations. But for a long time Delpech had no followers, until Dupuytren, in the last years of his life, operated for deformities of the nose.[66] Lisfranc,[67] and, more recently, Martinet, Jobert, Labat, and Blandin took up the work. With that chauvinism, so common among their countrymen, Labat and Blandin would have us believe that France was the country where plastic surgery flourished and developed its present stature. They would like to include Larrey as a rhinoplastic surgeon, because he pared and sutured old wounds of the nose from time to time ('rhinorrhaphy'), although it never crossed his

---

[58] See p. 52, n. 11.

[59] [Zeis admitted that he had not had full access to the English literature—see p. xiii, n. 11.]

[60] See p. 52, n. 13.

[61] J. F. Dieffenbach, *Chirurgische Erfahrungen, besonders über die Wiederherstellung zerstörter Theile des menschlichen Körpers nach neuen Methoden*, Berlin (1829–34). The sections of this dealing with the nose were translated by, and included in, J. S. Bushnan, *Surgical observations on the restoration of the nose*, London (1833).]

[62] [Jacques Mathieu Delpech (1772–1832), professor of surgery at Montpellier (1812). In 1832 he was shot by a patient on whom he had operated for a varicocele.]

[63] See p. 185, n. 2.

[64] J. M. Delpech, *Chirurgie clinique de Montpellier*, Vol. 2, Paris (1828).

[65] P. A. L. Labat, *De la rhinoplastie, art de restaurer ou de refaire complètement le nez*, Paris (1834). [Pierre Auguste Lèon Labat (1803–47), a great traveller, dedicated his book, the first on this subject in French, to the Viceroy of Egypt.]

[66] G. Dupuytren, Operations for the removal of various deformities at the Hospital of Lyons, *Lond. med. Gaz.* **5,** p. 799 (1830).]

[67] J. Lisfranc, Mémoire sur la rhinoplastie, *Bull. Sci. méd.* **12,** 238 (1827). [Rhinoplastic operation, performed by M. Lisfranc, followed by Death, *Lancet* **2,** 808 (1827–28).]

mind to take such an honour for himself.[68]

In Russia, Dr. Höfft carried out a rhinoplasty in Kursk by the Indian method, keeping strictly to Gräfe's technique.[69] Dybeck, in Warsaw, used Gräfe's method to replace one ala destroyed by syphilis.[70]

---

[68] [D. J. Larrey was a firm opponent of rhinoplasty: 'in our opinion it should not become part of surgery, Just as they decided in the 17th century.' *Clinique chirurgicale*, Vol. 2, Paris 18 (1829).]

[69] See p. 52, n. 21.

[70] See p. 44, n. 18.

3

THE REUNION OF COMPLETELY SEPARATED PARTS

The reunion of a completely separated part of the body does not really belong to plastic surgery, but it is so interesting that I may be forgiven for including it here, and all the more as the physiological and pathological conditions, under which a completely, or almost completely, severed part heals, are the same as those of transplanted skin, and may help to throw some light on the subject. Although the reunion of completely separated parts is attested by many indubitable examples, their success is too uncertain, the number of failures too great, and the conditions for healing still too little known to base a method of operation on them, or for a completely detached piece of skin to be used to repair a deformity. If the survival of such a piece could be predicted with the same certainty as that of a flap from the forehead, then plastic surgery would be in quite a different position from now, where the lack of healthy skin near a defect often makes all surgical help impossible.

Among the conditions for the reunion, the size of the piece seems to be particularly important. A small piece unites less well than a larger—a finger-tip less well than a whole phalanx, It seems as if the separated piece can maintain its own warmth and vitality for a time, until the circulation of blood is restored. But this also has its limits, and a very large part, such as an arm or a leg, will never unite, even with the most careful treatment. Montégre was the first to point out that union will fail if the reattachment is made too soon after the injury.[1] There is no doubt that both raw surfaces must be in close contact, without intervening clots, if there is to be primary healing. If there are clots, suppuration will always occur. If one waits until the bleeding has stopped, and the 'serous stage' is reached (usually 15–30 minutes), before attachment, the result will be better than if one is in too much of a hurry. Although it must seem that a nose that has been cut off with a

---

[1] [A.-F.-J. Montégre, editor of *Gaz. Santé. Paris* no. 7 (1817), was commenting on N. L. Lespagnol, Observation sur la réunion immédiate de l'extrémité d'un doigt qui avoit été entièrement coupée et séparée du corps, *J. Med. Pharm.* **39**, 273 (1817),—and other similar cases.]

sharp instrument would heal better than one that has been crushed or torn, it is surprising that noses that have been bitten off, fallen in mud or sand, found after a long search, and then washed and sutured in place, have still united.

EXPERIMENTS ON ANIMALS

The reunion of separated parts in animals does not help us much. It is known that the lower down the animal scale the greater the power of regeneration, so that it is not surprising that union in animals will be more successful than in man. Among the many experiments that have been carried out, I should mention the work of Dieffenbach (feathers, hairs, claws, and pieces of skin),[2] Du Hamel,[3] Gräfe,[4] Hunter (teeth and cock-spurs),[5] Merrem (bone),[6] and von Walther (bone).[7]

ATTEMPTS AT REUNION IN EARLIER TIMES

In earlier times the replacement of severed parts does not seem to have been attempted as often as it is nowadays, or people would have been all the sooner convinced that it is sometimes, although not always, successful. Lanfranc and many others expressed their disbelief in the possibility of reunion:

> many speak falsely of wounds of the nose, saying that it has been known for someone to carry his severed nose in his hand, and that it was afterwards replaced. This is completely false, because the vital spirit dies instantly.[8]

---

[2] J. F. Dieffenbach, Transplantationsversuche bei Thieren, *J. Chir. Augenheilk.* **6**, 122 (1824). [Attempts to transplant skin in pigeons, a hen, and a rabbit all failed.]

[3] H. L. Du Hamel, Recherches sur le réunion des plaies des arbres, sur la façon dont la greffe s'unit au sujet sur lequel on l'applique, sur la réunion des plaies des animaux, et quelques exemples de greffes appliquées sur des animaux, *Hist. Acad. r. Sci.* année 1746, p. 319 (Paris, 1751).

[4] C. F. von Gräfe, 'Gräfe misslangen alle (bis 1821) an Menschen und Thieren gemachten Versuch zur Transplantation ganz getrennter Theile, *J. Chir. Augenheilk.* **2**, 1 (1821).

[5] J. Hunter, *The natural history of the teeth*, London, p. 126 (1771).

[6] D. C. T. Merrem, *Animadversiones quaedam chirurgicae experimentis in animalibus factis*, Giessen, p. 16 (1810). [Successful healing of trepanned discs of bone in animals.]

[7] P. F. von Walther, Wiederanheilung der bei der Trepanation ausgebohrten Knochenscheibe, *J. Chir. Augenheilk.* **2**, 571 (1821).

[8] Lanfranc of Milan, *Chirurgia Magna*, Tract 2, Chapter 2, folio 177. In *Collectio Veneta*, Venice 1519.

This prejudice must have prevented them from attempting reunion, so that they would not have had the opportunity of seeing for themselves. It is surprising that they were so doubtful when, even today, laymen believe that a missing part can be replaced with hen's flesh.

When Fioravanti was in Africa, a Spanish nobleman had his nose cut off in a quarrel. Fioravanti picked it up, urinated on it to clean the sand off, and attached it to the stump, where it healed perfectly.[9] Blegny described a similar case in a soldier where there was hardly a scar to be seen.[10]

The most famous case is Garengeot's: two soldiers were quarrelling when one bit off the other's nose-tip, spat it in the gutter, and stamped on it. The owner picked it up, threw it into a barber-surgeon's shop, and ran after his opponent to get his revenge. The piece was washed at the well, and then warmed in wine; when the soldier came back, it was fixed to his nose with sticking-plaster, and by the fourth day it was healed.[11] Garengeot's report of this was widely disbelieved, and he received much abuse for it. Loubet had a similar case, but he was afraid that he would suffer the same fate as Garengeot, and so he kept it to himself.[12] Bossu, a surgeon in Arras, reported the case of a boy who had cut off his left thumb. Bossu attached the thumb, which the boy had brought in his pocket, to the bleeding stump, and it healed perfectly.[13] Ruddiman said that, in India, petty thieves are punished by having their noses cut off; the executioner then throws the piece in the fire, to prevent the victim reuniting it with its former site. The natives assured Ruddiman that this reunion had often been observed.[14] Sancassani tells the story of Gambacurta, a quack in Florence, who advertised her wound-salve by cutting a large piece out of her thigh, passing it round on a plate, and then replacing it, and dressing it with her ointment. It healed so quickly that the next evening no further dressing was needed.[15] Baronio also reported a charlatan in Rovate,

---

9 L. Fioravanti, [d. 1588] *Tesoro della vita humana*, Book 2, Venice, Chapter 45, p. 120 (1673).

10 N. de Blegny, *Zodiacus medico-gallicus*, Geneva, p. 72 (1682). [The nose had been struck off with a scimitar.]

11 R. J. C. Garengeot, *Traité des opérations de chirurgie*, Vol. 3, Paris, p. 55 (1731). [Full account in Nasal operation, *Lancet*, **1**, 233 (1823); and Carpue, *Two successful operations*, pp. 33–4.]

12 J. A. Loubet, *Traité des playes d'armes à feu*, Paris, p. 31 (1753).

13 Bossu, Sur la réunion de la troisiéme phalange du pouce après la section parfaite, *J. Méd. Pharm*, July, p. 78 (1770).

14 Carpue, *Two successful operations*, p. 61.

15 D. A. Sancassani, *Dilucidazioni fisico-mediche*, Vol. 1, Rome, p. 151 (1731).

who had an ointment that he called 'army balsam'. One market day in Cassano d'Adda he cut a large piece of skin from his arm, together with part of the radial muscle, showed it to the onlookers, and put it back in place with a dressing of his balsam. Eight days later the site of the wound could hardly be seen.[16]

REUNION IN RECENT TIMES

Balfour always tried to replace separated parts unless they were so big that this would have interfered with stopping the bleeding, A carpenter came to him, having cut off half his left index finger. Balfour sent for the finger, which was white and cold like a piece of candle, and joined it to the stump. When he saw the patient three weeks later, the finger was warm and had sensation, but the nail had fallen off. The testimony of three eye-witnesses puts this result beyond any doubt. Before this, Balfour had had a similar experience with his own son, and the favourable outcome encouraged him to make this attempt.[17] Carpue reported an observation by his friend, Sawrey, of a young Swede who had, as a boy, exchanged a piece of the skin of his arm with a friend, as a mark of indelible affection. The pieces of skin had united, and the marks were still recognizable.[18] Markiewicz reported that a tailor in Cracow was sitting at his window when the casement suddenly shut; his nose was cut off at the root by broken glass, and fell into the street two storeys below. A surgeon, who was a friend of the patient, arrived two hours later, searched for the nose, and replaced it. It was healed in a few days, and there was only a narrow red scar to be seen.[19]

Bünger's case[20]

This reconstruction of the nose with a completely detached piece of skin is more important for its physiological aspects—the reunion of a piece

---

[16] G. Baronio, *Degli innesti animali*, Milan, p. 28 (1804).

[17] W. Balfour, Two cases, with observations, demonstrative of the power of nature to reunite parts which have been, by accident, totally separated from the animal system, *Edinb. med. surg. J.* **10**, 421 (1814).

[18] Carpue, *Two successful operations*, p. 62.

[19] R. Markiewicz, Nachricht über die Anheilung einer zwei Stunden lang völlig abgetrennten Nase, *J. Chir. Augenheilk.* **7**, 538 (1825).

[20] H. C. Bünger, Gelungener Versuch einer Nasenbildung aus einem völlig getrennten Hautstück aus dem Beine, *J. Chir, Augenheilk.* **4**, 569 (1823). [Heinrich Christian Bünger (1782–1842) was professor of anatomy at Marburg (1815–40).]

of skin that had been detached for a long time—than as an operation to repair the face.

A woman aged 33, with lupus for 15 years, had lost the lower part of her nose; the disease was still active in various parts of her face. Bünger had excised some of these areas, which had improved her appearance, and he decided to remove the whole of the remaining diseased area. But the forehead was not large enough to replace this, and he wished to save the patient a scar on her forehead. Her cheeks were already scarred, and they could not provide enough skin. He considered the Italian method, but it would have been very difficult to attach the flap near the angle of the eye. He also dismissed the idea of taking the skin from another person, because of the difficulty of keeping two people joined together, even for a short time. Finally he decided on the most hazardous method of all—taking a completely detached piece of skin from a distant part of her body. The only thing in its favour was that, if it failed, a scar on a distant site would not be so disfiguring. Bünger selected the front of the top of her thigh; if he had taken the skin from the buttock it would have been uncomfortable for her to sit or lie after the operation, He had this area beaten with a strap until it was deeply red and swollen.

Bünger started the operation by excising the diseased facial skin, and preparing the defect on the nose, but it took him an hour to get the bleeding more or less under control. The piece of skin required was four inches long and three inches wide. Only when it had been completely detached did Bünger trim it to shape, and remove the fat. The piece of skin in his hand was chalk-white, and had long since cooled, as the facial wound was still bleeding. It was another hour and a half before he decided to go ahead, rather in the hope that the piece of skin and the sutures would stop the bleeding. The number of sutures is not recorded. The skin was the shape of a nose, but deathly white. The dressing was of very fine lint and linen, and, to warm the skin, Bünger asked her to cup her hands over it and breathe out frequently. The next day her face was red and swollen; the nose was white, but with no discoloured areas. The wound on the thigh was very painful. On the third day, to Bünger's and Professor Ullmann's[21] great surprise, the skin was bright red, shiny, and swollen; only a narrow strip of the part forming the columella and ala showed a suspicious blueish tinge. Healing was thus taking place from the surface, and not from the

[21] [Christoph Ullmann, Zeis' predecessor in the chair of surgery in Marburg, assisted at the operation.]

margins. For fear of gangrene, several sutures were removed, and the flap was dressed with decoctions of china and sabina.[22] On the fourth day, the blueish areas had spread; all sutures were removed. The skin was firmly adherent to the bed, but the margins were not united. By the evening, small blisters had appeared in the blue areas. The gangrene did not extend further, but became demarcated by laudable pus, so that the columella and ala were sloughed off, The margins healed by granulation in five weeks. Small pustules formed on the skin, and the thickened epidermis was shed three times, under which a new layer had always developed. Finally, small fine hairs sprouted, as would be found on the thigh. The piece of skin from the thigh remained in good condition on the face, only distinguished by its paler colour. Sunlight, localized to this area, should turn it brown. One year later, Bünger excised a patch of disease on the upper lip, and then carried out a rhinoplasty by Gräfe's method. The skin from the arm united with the skin of the thigh to make the nose-tip and the columella, but the part for the ala failed to unite, and had to be reconstructed later from the cheek.[23]

Von Walther's case[24]

This is an even more important case.

A healthy young man aged 22, while staying in Bonn, had the lower part of his nose cut off with a sabre, losing the tip, half the right ala, and one third of the left ala, with parts of both nasal bones. The bleeding was very severe, and did not stop until the man fainted. The nose lay on the floor for five minutes, and it was frequently trodden on in the confusion. Dr Alt, who was present, found the piece, cleaned it, and reattached it with four sutures and sticking-plaster. On the fifth day it seemed to be healthy and uniting well. But two days later it was discoloured, stinking, and covered with a dry scab. The edges began to separate, and exuded thin pus. Von Walther thought that the attachment had failed, but, as the sutures were still holding, he left the part in place, and ordered frequent dressings of a decoction of china[25] and spirits of camphor. The skin contracted, and the flow of pus increased

---

[22] [Irritants—Peruvian bark and savin (*Juniperus sabina*).]

[23] [See also H. May, Successful attempt of reconstruction of a nose from a completely separated piece of skin from the leg, *Plastic reconstr. Surg.* **44**, 569 (1969).

[24] P. F. von Walther, Wiederanheilung einer ganz abgehauenen Nase, *J. Chir. Augenheilk.* **7**, 521 (1825).

[25] [See n. 22 above.]

and improved in quality. Some sutures were left until the eighteenth day, when the upper end had separated completely. Von Walther lifted the scab off, and was amazed to find that the whole raw surface of the nose was covered with a layer of the most beautiful granulations. The parts of the scab that had not separated were excised.

Thus the part had not become gangrenous in full-thickness, but only in its outer layer. The deeper layer was alive, and had united with the stump of the nose. There was a small hole in the middle, through which one could look into the nasal cavity. Here there had been full-thickness loss, but this area was furthest from all nutrient supply, and also had no underlying support. The raw surface was dressed with cerate,[26] and it quickly healed; the hole in the middle closed spontaneously. Six months later the nose had not contracted, but was rather swollen, red like scar tissue, with a wrinkled surface, and many blood-vessels; gradually it became paler.

The gangrene of the outer layer would have deceived most surgeons, and they would have given up all hope that the nose could be saved. But von Walther's deep knowledge of physiology, and his skilful management, won the day, and spared the patient a hideous deformity.

Hoffacker's cases

Hoffacker[27] reported 13 successful cases of reunion of completely separated parts. He noted that there was nearly always gross discolouration at the first dressing, and then, as in von Walther's case, that there would be desquamation of the outer layer of the skin, under which good granulations were sprouting.[28] Braun made similar observations.[29]

There have been so many cases where parts, mainly of the face, but also arms and hands, have been incompletely severed, remaining attached by a narrow pedicle, and have reunited, that no one now

[26] [Lard and white wax.]

[27] [Gottlieb Wilhelm Hoffacker (1787–1844) was the most famous '*Paukdoctor*' (surgeon to the student duellists) of his day. He had unrivalled experience of the replacement of parts of the face, completely detached by sabre cuts, in the student duelling clubs of the university of Heidelberg. No other surgeon had so many cases of successful reunion—see *Lancet* **1**, 340 (1830–31).]

[28] G. W. Hoffacker, Beobachtungen über die Anheilung abgehauener Stücke der Nase und Lippen, *Heidelb. klin. Annln.* **4**, 232 (1828).

[29] J. A. Braun, 'Wiederanheilung eines gänzlich abgeschnittenen Fingers', *Magazin ges. Heilk.* **14** (1823), 112.

doubts this possibility. They are more common than complete separation, and it is easier to explain how their nourishment is maintained. There is no need for me to give a list of them here.

Dieffenbach's experiments

A woman aged 30 was anaesthetic down the whole of the left side of her body, so that she could be pricked, burned, or pinched without feeling anything. For 24 hours before the operation, the skin of her arm was rubbed with spirit until it was red and hot. A piece of skin one-and-a-half inches in diameter was cut from the reddened part of the inner side of her forearm; she only felt a tickling sensation. Then a piece of the same size was cut from the outer side of her arm. The pieces were transposed, and held in place with sticking-plaster and a bandage. Both pieces contracted, and became blueish-white. When the dressings were removed on the sixth day, the piece on the inner side was dissolved in good thick pus. On the outer side, more than half had turned to pus, but the rest was like a rounded mass of granulations, attached to the bed by reddish cellular tissue. Unfortunately, Dieffenbach pulled this off by mistake, thinking that it was granulation tissue; but streaks of blood from the wound showed clearly that union had taken place.[30]

REUNION OF BONE

Van Meek'ren has recorded the story by the monk, Kraanwinkel, that a Russian nobleman, who had lost a piece of his skull, had it replaced by a piece taken from a dog's skull. For this, the Russian was excommunicated, and could only redeem himself by having the piece of bone removed.[31]

But there is good evidence that detached pieces of bone, particularly the bony discs from trepanning, can heal back into the same place. Von Walther experimented by replacing a trepanned piece of bone in a dog. When the dog was killed a year later, the trepanned disc appeared whiter than the rest of the skull, and there was hardly a trace of callus to be seen. The question was whether the piece was living, or whether it was simply held in place mechanically. This was answered by the case of a 36-year-old bricklayer in whom a trepanned piece of bone, to which

[30] J. F. Dieffenbach, Ueberpflanzung völlig getrennter Hautstücke bei einer Frau und Wiederanheilung einer grösstentheils abgehauenen Wange, *J. Chir. Augenheilk.* **6**, 482 (1824).

[31] J. van Meek'ren, *Observationes medico-chirurgicae*, Amsterdam, p. 6 (1682).

the periosteum had been left attached, was replaced. The wound did not heal, and continued to suppurate for several months. The freely mobile piece of bone could be felt in the depths. After three months von Walther thought that he should remove it, and was not a little surprised to find, instead of the complete bony disc, only a thin jagged piece of bone. This was a fragment of the outer table, roughened on its under surface, which looked like a sequestrum. The hole in the skull was completely closed, so that the inner table had united, and the movements of the brain were no longer apparent. This shows that the trepanned disc must have been alive, and that the inner table was not just being held in place mechanically.[32]

REUNION OF TEETH

Replacement of teeth has often been tried. A French dentist, Capron, in the middle of the eighteenth century, is said to have replaced a nobleman's tooth with one from a Savoyard; this operation was often attempted in England at that time.[33] Wiesmann extracted and reinserted a tooth in a dog, fixing it to the neighbouring teeth. When the dog was killed seven weeks later, he found that the tooth was attached to the gum, and that a number of small vessels were running to the socket, with one injected vessel entering the tooth itself.[34] Fauchard even demonstrated the fixation of a dead tooth into a socket, which functioned as well as the rest of the teeth.[35] But this, of course, can only have been mechanical retention. Minding's recent attempts to replace roots of teeth, after they had been extracted and had crowns screwed on to them, should not be repeated, for the crowns broke off, and the roots were resorbed.[36]

---

32 [See n. 7 above.]

33 J. H. F. Wiesmann, *De coalitu partium a reliquo corpore prorsus disjunctarum*, Leipzig, p. 19 (1824).

34 Ibid. p. 25.

35 P. Fauchard, *Le chirurgien dentiste, ou traité des dents*, Vol. 2 Paris, p. 182 (1728).

36 J. Minding, Ein Beitrag zur Chirurgia curtorum. In J. C. A. Clarus und J. Radius, *Beiträge zur praktische Heilkunde*, Vol. 3, Leipzig, p. 194 (1836).

4

THE ITALIAN METHOD OF RECONSTRUCTION

The main methods of reconstruction are, from the less to the more perfect, Tagliacozzi's (the Italian), Gräfe's modification of this (the German), and the Indian.

A summary of Tagliacozzi's writings on *chirurgia curtorum* is given here to show the state of plastic surgery several centuries ago, and how accurate his observations were. It is essential to understand his technique, because his method is still practicable; with minor modifications it has been used in recent times, and will sometimes be needed in the future. But the Indian method will always be preferred, as it is easier and more certain of success. Nevertheless, there are a few patients in whom skin near the defect cannot be used, so that it has to be transplanted from a distance. Tagliacozzi was only concerned with the replacement of noses, lips, or ears. There is no mention of any other parts of the body in his book, but there are two cases of repair of a nose which had had a piece sliced out of the bridge.[1] He regarded the lip as more difficult than the nose, as it needs a larger piece of skin; even today cheiloplasty is more difficult than rhinoplasty. He reconstructed the ear, not with skin from the arm, but with local skin, like the Indian method, which he never used for the nose. He was convinced of the value of his work, and anxious to make it more widely known, but he recognized the imperfections in a reconstructed nose: that it could be too small, a different colour from the rest of the face, too soft, lacking sensation, hairy, and with contracted nostrils.[2] Some of these problems still occur today, but it can be expected that results will be improved by the further development of the Indian method and the discovery of new techniques.

Tagliacozzi showed himself to be a careful physician by his attention to the general condition of the patient before operation.[3] He stressed that, if the deformity was not due to injury, but to underlying disease,

---

[1] Tagliacozzi, *de curtorum*, Vol. 1, Chapter 23.

[2] Ibid. Vol. 1, Chapter 24.

[3] Ibid. Vol. 2, Chapter 2.

such as syphilis, preliminary treatment should be undertaken, and the operation postponed until all disease was eradicated. The greater virulence of syphilis in his time, which was much closer to the origin of the disease than now, and the lack of systematic treatment, made this advice all the more important. He gave a list of purges and prescriptions, with the warning that the liver should not be over-stimulated. Preliminary blood-lettings were only occasionally necessary. The rest of his instructions are simply those for any surgical operation.

TAGLIACOZZI'S METHOD OF RHINOPLASTY

The piece of skin for reconstruction of the nose had to be carefully chosen. It should not have large blood-vessels running through it, and, when raised, it should not expose important structures; hairy skin was also unsuitable. But, most particularly, the part from which the skin was taken had to be easily brought up to the stump of the nose, so that it would not put too great a strain on the patient to be held in this position until union had occurred. On all these counts, the skin of the upper arm was best for rhinoplasty; the scar that it left was less of a disability on the left arm, which was therefore preferred.

At least six operations were needed:

(1) raising the flap as a bridge of skin;
(2) dividing one end of the bridge, so that it remained attached to the arm by only one pedicle;
(3) the principal operation—suturing the flap to the stump of the nose;
(4) separating the flap from the arm;
(5) forming the nostrils and the columella;
(6) suturing the columella to the upper lip.

The first operation

The patient lay on a bed with his arm on a pillow, so that it was not injured by involuntary movements due to the pain. (Tagliacozzi warned of the danger of injuring the veins, but it is not as easy to avoid them as when the flap is raised in one stage, and the surgeon can see where he is cutting). The skin over the biceps, on the inner side of the left upper arm, was lifted in a longitudinal fold that had to be wide enough, after it had contracted by a quarter or a third, to make the nose. This fold was held in Tagliacozzi's special forceps, and separated from the underlying tissues with a scalpel, so that it formed a bridge.

The inexperienced surgeon should mark the incisions beforehand. A piece of linen, exactly the size of the wound, was laid under the flap. If the piece was too long, its edges would have to be rolled, and would cause unnecessary pain; if it was too narrow, it would allow the flap to become partially reattached. For the dressing, Tagliacozzi recommended olive-oil and turpentine, and in the winter, when the skin was colder, an even more stimulating ointment. The dressing was left until the fourth day, and then, when pus had formed, was changed daily to encourage scarring on the under-surface of the flap.
flap.

All his other instructions will be omitted here, as his prescriptions are very complicated and too stimulating. It is to be hoped that modern surgery, with its simpler, milder remedies, will never go back to the quackery of the Middle Ages.

The second operation

When contraction had made the flap thicker, without interfering with its nutrition, the third side could be divided—about 14 days after the first operation. If the flap was destined for the nose or the upper lip, the upper end nearer the axilla was divided; for the lower lip, the lower end nearer the elbow was divided, so that there was no need to twist the flap before it was attached. If the flap was the right size, the incision was made straight across over a grooved director; if it was too small, the incision was curved. Tagliacozzi advised that it was better to make the flap too big than too small: 'for it is essential to be prepared for all contingencies.'[4] (This is a rule that, even now, cannot be stressed too strongly, especially in reconstruction from the forehead, where the fear of disfigurement means that the flap is often too small, and the operation is spoiled.) A dressing was put under the flap to prevent it becoming reattached to its bed. Tagliacozzi often noticed that pustules erupted on and around the flap, which delayed the next stage, and made the patient scratch, so as to draw blood.[5] (It seems likely that this was caused by his over-stimulating ointments.) Another complication was a thin, foul discharge which ulcerated the surrounding skin. The greatest cleanliness was therefore essential, and the flap was to be kept from contact with the skin by dressings.

Tagliacozzi compared the changes in a flap to the ages of man: when the flap had just been raised, and was still soft and moist, he called this

[4] Ibid. Vol. 2, Chapter 8.
[5] Ibid. Vol. 2, Chapter 9, p. 27.

its 'childhood' (*pueritia*). It needed great care because it was now only nourished from one end, and ulcers, inflammation, and even gangrene could occur. Next came 'youth' (*adolescentia*), as the flap became dryer and firmer, and the under-surface began to scar over, starting at the edges and the tip, and spreading towards the pedicle. When this was complete, the flap had reached 'manhood' (*aetas virilis*), which was the best time for suturing it to the nose. If this was delayed, the flap contracted too much, and the hardening scar-tissue reduced the flow of fluid through the pedicle. This was 'old age' (*senectus*), which left only a pale, dry, wrinkled, unhealthy flap.

The third operation

If the patient was in good health when his flap had reached 'manhood'—usually about the fourteenth day after the second operation—the flap could be sutured to the nose. The morning of a fine day was chosen for the operation, The patient's head and beard were shaved, so that the cap for securing the arm would sit firmly on his head, and vermin would not be retained under it. If the patient had not opened his bowels, he was given an enema. He then put on trousers, a leather jacket, and a cap to which the straps for the arm would be attached. A cobbler was present at the operation in case alterations were needed. The surgeon was to set out the instruments in advance: straight and curved knives, forceps, scissors, needles, thread, and linen.[6] (Tagliacozzi even mentioned that the surgeon should remove his clothes, so that he would be more comfortable.) The patient sat on a stool with a back-rest, as this was most convenient for the surgeon. (Tagliacozzi did not think it necessary to mark out the incisions, as the ink only gets washed off by the blood.)

The operation started by freshening the stump of the nose, in the way that one would graft a tree, i.e. the incision was not made at right angles, but obliquely, through the skin, taking away more of the epidermis than the dermis, to prevent overgrowth of granulations which would lead to prominent scars.[7] Then a drawing was made of the shape of the new nose, and transferred to the flap, so that any excess could be cut away. This was the most important step in the operation. (Tagliacozzi urged most strongly that the flap should not be made too small.) Then the incisions were adjusted so that the edges of the flap and the stump of the nose matched exactly. During the operation, a cloth was wrapped round the patient's forehead, to which the sutures

[6] Ibid. Vol. 2, Chapter 11, p. 33.

[7] Ibid. Vol. 2, Chapter 12, p. 39.

and needles were fastened so that they did not get tangled. The sutures had to be long enough to reach from the arm to the nose, before these had been brought together, without tension and without pulling out.

To ensure that the parts were accurately apposed, the line of sutures on the flap formed the arc of a smaller circle *b* than on the stump *a*, so that they lay like the radii of a circle *c,c,c* [Fig. 2]. The central suture was inserted first, and they should all be an equal distance apart. When all the sutures had been inserted, the patient was returned to bed. The sutures were then tied, starting with the one in the middle. One assistant held the patient's hand firmly to his head, another held the elbow, and a third brought the flap to the stump. The surgeon tied the sutures, cut the ends, put lint smeared with white of egg in the nostrils, and dressed the wounds.

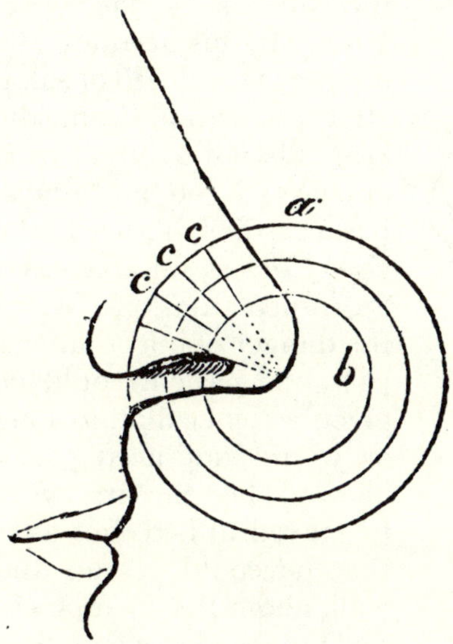

Fig. 2

Then the straps were fitted [Fig. 3]. The first ran from the chest to the elbow, and along the forearm to the head, *abc*. The second started at the shoulder, and ran under the axilla to pull the shoulder towards the mid-line, *dd*. The third started from the first at the elbow, went to the right temple and was fastened there to the cap to prevent sideways movements of the head, *e*. The fourth ran from the elbow to the right side of the chest, *fg*. The fifth, *h*, encircled the wrist and the third band, and held the hand to the head.

The after-care needed the greatest attention to ensure that the wound edges remained exactly together. On the outside the sutures were supported by sticking-plaster, but it was more difficult to get apposition on the inside, and the moisture of the nasal mucus always interfered with healing. (Tagliacozzi was quite right to note the poor adhesive inflammation of mucous membrane, and its tendency to form pus.) To prevent infection in the stitch-holes, Tagliacozzi recommended keeping the wound clean, smearing it with myrrh and frankincense, and changing the dressing frequently. To do this, the strap from the elbow to the right temple was loosened, and the arm was held by an assistant. Union occurred by the third day, or, in unfavourable conditions, the fourth–fifth days. Sutures were removed from the places that were driest and most completely united. This was usually at the top, where there was least disturbance from the flow of mucus. All the sutures should not be removed at once. Tagliacozzi sometimes left some of them until the seventh day, but to wait longer was harmful because the tracks became infected, and left unsightly scars.

He divided the flap towards the end of the third week.[8] This was much earlier than his predecessors, who waited cautiously until the fortieth day. Once the flap had united, he felt no further anxiety about the success of the operation. (By his account, the danger of the death of a flap after separation from the arm was not as great as it appears to be nowadays; perhaps the fault lies in the choice of less suitable cases for transplantation.) When the danger of infection was past, the patient could be given a richer diet, as long as it did not need to be chewed. For the first week he stayed in bed, but after that he could get up and walk about the room. Gentle purgatives ensured a bowel action at least every other day. All excitement was to be avoided.

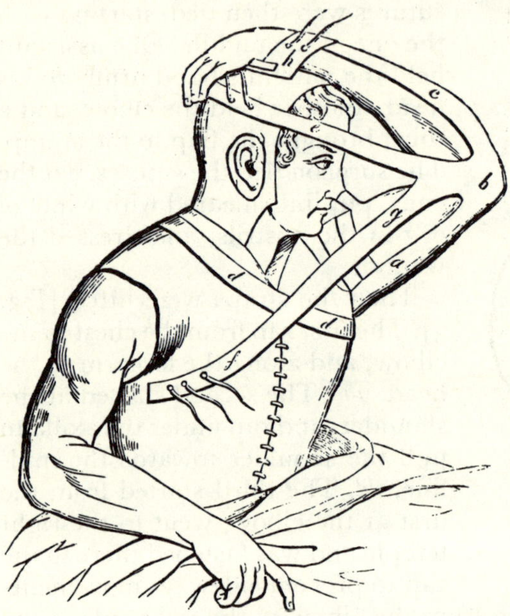

Fig. 3

But things did not always go so smoothly. Tagliacozzi gave as the first complication the growth of proud flesh and gaping of the suture line. The next was pain in the region of the shoulder-blade, due to the cramped position of the arm, and the harness pulling the shoulder-blade away from the midline; pain in the shoulder itself was less common. There was little that could be done about it, for loosening the straps would endanger the flap. Sometimes there was also pain in the wrist, and it was important to see that the cap was well made, with no stitching where the hand lay. Without moving the arm, lint or cotton wool could be laid carefully under the wrist. The patient might also be

---

[8] Ibid. Vol. 2, Chapter 15.

tormented by thirst, sleeplessness, or pain in the kidneys. For the thirst, Tagliacozzi advised that slices of melon should be held in the mouth, and, for the pain in the kidneys, application of cow's or human milk and *ung. galeni refrigerans*.[9]

The fourth operation

As soon as the flap had united, it was separated from the arm. Union was always complete in the course of a week. Tagliacozzi, although quicker than his predecessors, waited another week or more, regarding the twentieth day as the latest for the separation. The arm was held by an assistant, and the base of the flap was divided.

Then came the after-care of the flap, bringing the arm down, and dressing the wound on the arm. The surgeon dealt with the first of these, and left the other two to his assistants. There was no need to be anxious if the flap became pale and cold, for it would recover with proper treatment. This appearance was the natural result of the sudden cutting-off of the nourishment through the base of the flap, which would continue until blood started to circulate through the scar. Other parts of the body could become cold and white in very cold weather, without dying. A flap always retained some of its vital warmth, and it could be quickly revived by speeding the flow of blood to it with warm compresses. An assistant dressed the wound on the arm with white of egg and a bandage. Bringing the arm down was very hard for the patient, and had to be done gradually. While one assistant saw to this, another prepared a pillow for the arm to lie on.

If the flap was too big, so that it was not all needed for the nose, the excess should not be set back in the arm. Tagliacozzi recognized that this was difficult to do, and simply left a useless lump on the arm.[10] It was better to divide the flap close to the arm, and leave as much as possible on the nose, in case there was further contraction. If it was still too big, it was never too late to remove the excess. But as soon as it was certain how much had to be removed, this was done, for the excess hung down and interfered with eating.

The fifth operation

About 14 days after separating the flap from the arm, the nostrils and columella were fashioned. During this time, drying ointments were used on the inner surface to promote scarring, and the flap was washed

---

[9] [Galena—lead sulphide.]

[10] Ibid. Vol. 2, Chapter 15, p. 55.

with wine and musk to stimulate it. This operation was the opportunity to make the nose beautiful.[11] The nose should be one-third of the length of the face, and the flap was measured for this with compasses. If part of one ala remained, this was the guide for the new one, taking care to make the nostrils symmetrical. The incisions for the nostrils were made along previously drawn curved lines, continued as straight incisions to form the columella; the latter incisions were made vertically through the skin, so as not to weaken the columella. The incisions for the nostrils were oblique, so that the free margins of the alae became covered with epidermis and not with granulations and scar-tissue. Quills were put in the nostrils, and the columella, which was to be sutured later, was held in place with a dressing. The columella must be very broad, as it would contract, and it had to support the tip of the nose.

After 3–4 weeks the patient could go outside, but he had to be careful of inclement weather. The suture of the columella to the upper lip was better postponed, so that granulations could be removed from the inside of the nose. Tagliacozzi stated that, if the columella was attached at once, it would pull the nose-tip down by its contraction; it should therefore only be sutured at 38–60 days.

The sixth operation

If a piece of the old columella remained, Tagliacozzi sutured the new one to it. If it was completely missing, he used his special forceps to lift the lip away from the upper jaw, so that it could be incised. He did not use a knife, because of the mobility of the columella, and because scissors caused less pain in the very sensitive upper lip.[12] After incising the upper lip, the columella was freshened, shortened if necessary, and attached with one interrupted suture which was left until the fourth day.

After-treatment

When all the operative stages had been completed, there was still a long time to be spent in shaping the new nose. The poor nutrition of the flap at first made it contract, but this gradually improved. Fourteen–twenty-one days after suture of the columella, tubes, which were flattened where they rested against the columella, were placed in the nose. These were best made of lead to prevent granulations; later they could

[11] Ibid. Vol. 2, Chapter 16, p. 56.

[12] 'We seize the parts quickly, and make an incision at a single stroke, as quickly as possible, giving not the slightest forewarning of the pain.' op. cit. p. 62.

be of gold or silver, and the same for the splint that went over the nose. This splint (*tectorium*) was held on the face by bands, and the tubes were attached to it. It had to have the shape of a good-looking nose, so that this could be transmitted to the new nose during the two years that it was worn continuously. If the nose was still pale and discoloured, it should be exposed to the sun for short periods, without harming the head and the rest of the face. Prominent scars were excised and re-sutured; if they were less severe, they could be smoothed out by binding on lead plates.

These, briefly, are Tagliacozzi's instructions for rhinoplasty, based on his wide experience. All his writings show him to have been a true observer of nature, so that it is unbelievable that, for a time, his doctrine was regarded as pure fabrication. This was the reason why his operation was not copied. But he had described it in the greatest detail, and there was certainly no lack of opportunity to practise it. Perhaps he would have had more success in persuading other surgeons, if he had included case histories in his book; this was not the custom in his time, although it is overdone nowadays. But to show their value, here is one of von Gräfe's cases:

VON GRÄFE'S FIRST ITALIAN RHINOPLASTY[13]

Here he kept strictly to Tagliacozzi's technique.[14] In 1814, a soldier lost the whole of the cartilaginous part of his nose from a sabre-cut. Gräfe did the first operation on 8 May 1816, raising a double-pedicled flap six inches long by four inches wide. This was followed by severe inflammation, and the flap did not regain its normal colour for four weeks. On 7 June the upper end of the flap was divided, causing the patient severe pain; there was only slight bleeding. The flap became pale and cold, with diminished sensation. It contracted markedly, and became inflamed again, with much exudate, which was thin at first, but gradually changed to the more favourable thick yellow pus. The patient's arm had now lain so long on the pillow that he could not lift it without pain.

In August the wound on the arm was nearly healed, and scar-tissue was beginning to form on the flap. By September the flap was much smaller and wrinkled. Its under-surface was not completely healed until October. Gräfe described the position on 18 October:[15] the wound on the arm was covered with thin blueish scar tissue. The flap had shrunk to one-third of its original size. The skin was wrinkled and

[13] See p. 14, n. 50.
[14] Gräfe, *Rhinoplastik*, p. 105.
[15] Ibid, p. 114.

covered with a profuse growth of hair, but of normal colour. The under-surface was markedly concave, and the edges were so far curved round that the skin was doubled, and, in the middle, was covered with epidermis which only differed from the rest in its thinness and lack of hair. After the flap had been attached to the nose, the pieces of skin that were removed showed that the subcutaneous tissue was greatly increased, and had changed, so that its cut surface was milky, thickened, but not hard, and interspersed with small fatty nodules. Only a little blood oozed out, and the whole tissue had become like the cartilage of the ear or the tip of the nose. Gräfe admitted that the flap had already reached the stage that Tagliacozzi called 'old age', and that he had therefore delayed its attachment too long; this should have been carried out six weeks earlier, when the flap was still in 'manhood'. But the stages in Gräfe's case were much slower than Tagliacozzi had described, and this is probably due to the difference in the climate in the north and the south, rather than to the condition of the patient, for he was young and healthy.

On 19 October the flap was attached to the stump of the nose. The bony septum projected too far, and this was reduced with bone-cutters. Parts of the alae remained, and these were preserved. Six sutures were used, which were tightened with ligature-rods,[16] because the much thicker skin of the flap tended to overlap the thinner skin of the nose. After putting on the harness, the patient was taken back to bed. That evening he complained of pain in his shoulder and forearm, and his pulse was thin and rather fast. He was relieved by a dose of opium, and massage with liniment. Acidulous drinks were given with a spoon. The next day the flap was red and swollen, with exudation of coagulating lymph. On the third day the redness and swelling had increased, the suture-line was moist, and the scar on the arm had broken open in several places; the left cheek, where the arm was in contact, was red and excoriated. The arm and the face were dressed with lead lotion. The pain in the shoulder, which had increased, started to improve. By the eighth day the right side was firmly united, but union was less secure on the bridge of the nose and the left side; the sutures, which were cutting in, were removed, and the stitch-holes were dabbed with *Balsam, Commendatoris*.[17]

At the end of October the suture-lines on the bridge and the lower part of the left side were still gaping. The flap was very thick, and raised above the surface of the nose. Its appearance had improved with the increased vitality from its new attachment. On 1 November, 14 days

[16] See p. 101.

[17] [Tinct. benz. co.]

after its attachment to the nose, the flap was separated from the arm. Only a little blood oozed from the cut surface, and not very much more from the arm. The flap immediately became pale and cold. The wounds were dressed, and the nose was wrapped in cotton wool.

The next day the flap had returned to normal colour and temperature, but it was very swollen. Over the next few days the lower end of the flap, which had been turned up, began to sink into its intended place, touching the upper lip, and was held there with sticking-plaster. The gaping suture-line on the bridge of the nose did not heal until the beginning of December, after two applications of the actual cautery. On 1 January 1817 the gaping incision in the left ala was freshened and re-sutured. This finally healed, so that the next stage could then be carried out. As so much time had passed, and the flap had become as hard as cartilage, Gräfe did not think it necessary to keep exactly to Tagliacozzi's plan of making the nostrils and attaching the columella in two separate operations. This combined operation, on 5 February, was followed by considerable inflammation, and the flap became very swollen, but healing was satisfactory, and the sutures were removed after two days.

From this time on, the patient began to notice increased feeling in the flap. The temperature of the flap was the same as the rest of the face; in cold wind it became colder more quickly, and developed goose-flesh. There was a strong growth of hair, and the pallor of the flap contrasted with the colour of the cheeks. Gräfe subsequently cut away the projections formed by the thickening of the flap, with flat sweeps of the knife; the patient, who previously had no sensation in the flap, now experienced a little pain. When this was healed, lead tubes and a compression splint were applied, and the nose was kept wrapped in cotton wool. By April the shape of the nose had greatly improved, and its colour was more like the rest of the face, although it was always kept covered. It was also remarkable how the skin of the stump of the nose was drawn towards the flap from all sides, so that it appeared to be much longer, and the flap to be relatively smaller. By the end of April the nose looked as if it had been rough hewn, but it conformed reasonably well to the character of the face.

At the end of this report Gräfe expressed the hope that the new nose would, in time, come to match the face even more, and to resemble a real nose. The final result is not known, but such a hope seems unlikely to be fulfilled, Many flaps, even though they look satisfactory immediately after the operation, have, after several years, contracted so much that their appearance, although not to be compared with the original deformity, still constitutes a considerable disfigurement.

5

GRÄFE'S MODIFICATION OF THE ITALIAN METHOD—THE GERMAN METHOD

Tagliacozzi had already shortened his predecessors' method, leaving less time between the operative stages. But he advised against attaching the flap immediately it had been raised, because of the danger of inflammation, and because shrinkage could easily make it too small.[1] Reneaume de la Garanne, without ever doing a rhinoplasty himself, suggested that Tagliacozzi's procedure could be shortened by combining the first two stages.[2] Gräfe, after following Tagliacozzi's instructions in one case,[3] went even further, and not only raised the flap, but attached it to the nose, in one operation. He called this the 'German' modification of Tagliacozzi's method, and it is the origin of the concept of using a freshly raised and unscarred flap for reconstruction. His aims were: first, to take a smaller piece of skin from the arm, as there would be no need to allow as much for shrinkage as with the Italian method; secondly, to transplant a piece of skin that would match the thickness of the skin of the face, for, by waiting too long, the increased thickness of the flap prevents exact suturing, and the two edges are not level; and thirdly, to reduce the whole time to six weeks, and thus combine the advantages of the Indian method with the Italian, without, however, putting the patient at risk by laying bare the skull, and leaving him with a disfiguring scar on the forehead.

Gräfe's method is suitable for patients in good general health, with strong, mobile, well-nourished skin on the arm. If this is not the case, the flap must not be moved without waiting for it to contract. For several days before the operation the skin of the arm is rubbed with spirit. The patient should wear the harness from time to time, so that he gets used to the fixation of his arm to his head; he should sometimes sleep in it. Gräfe does not think it necessary to shave the head. Before

---

[1] Tagliacozzi, *de curtorum*, Vol. 2, Chapter 10, p. 32.

[2] See p. 12, n. 32.

[3] See p. 35.

the start of the operation the patient puts on the special jacket, but care must be taken not to get it splashed with blood. Gräfe gives detailed instructions for the equipment and for the duties of the assistants. The equipment consists of:

(1) clay or wax to make a model, a piece of paper, scissors to cut out the pattern, colour-varnish that will not wash off,[4] a fine brush, and a pencil;

(2) sharp instruments, including bone-cutters for the bony septum;

(3) material for controlling bleeding;

(4) 10–12 long doubled linen threads with a needle at each end, the little rods of ivory or boxwood (devised by him to put under the sutures to bring the skin edges level), and sticking-plaster; plaster;

(5) dressings and fixation materials;

(6) refreshment for the patient.

A model is made of the nose, and the measurements are transferred to a piece of paper, adding one-quarter in all dimensions to allow for shrinkage. This is cut out in soft leather, which is used to find the best place on the arm for the flap. Gräfe even marks out the points of suture beforehand, on the flap as well as on the stump of the nose, by cutting small holes in the paper pattern, and marking the arm through them.

The operation starts by freshening the stump of the nose. Tagliacozzi incised the mucosa first, then the skin, and then removed the strip in between, which seems unnecessarily complicated. Gräfe altered this by excising the margins in one stage, which is easier, and leaves the edges more even.

Then the flap is raised on the arm [Fig. 4]. The edges *a b c*, which are to be sutured immediately to the stump of the nose, keep to the shape of the pattern. But the columella (*d*), which will be attached later, must be considerably larger, as in Tagliacozzi's method, not only to allow for contraction, but also because it lies in the pedicle on which the nourishment of the flap depends. The sutures are passed from within outwards through the stump of the nose and the flap at the marked points. It is easier, when the flap is taken from the left arm, to start on the left side. Before the sutures are tightened, the wound on the arm is covered with a dressing well smeared with grease to stop it sticking, The arm is now brought close to the face, and the sutures are drawn together with

[4] *vernicis succini* [varnish] four parts, *fulig. opt. puriss.* [soot] one part.

ligature-rods. These make the task much easier, for there is little room between the arm and the face for ordinary knots; but they have the great disadvantage that, however carefully they are fixed to the face, their weight makes them pull on the sutures and the flap. Gräfe himself has stopped using them for this reason. He also recommends putting the sutures closer together.[5] Then the dressings are applied, with light packing in the nose, gauze covered with ointment on the raw surface of the flap, and narrow strips soaked in *Commandeur-balsam*[6] on the suture-line. The flap and the nose are covered with cotton wool to keep them warm. Finally the harness is applied to hold the arm to the head.

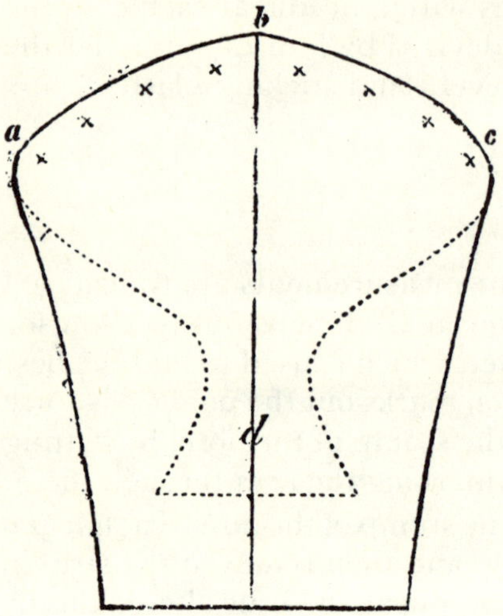

Fig. 4

Gräfe found that, to keep the arm still, Tagliacozzi's harness had to be pulled so tight that it caused considerable pain. Also, the straps from the arm to the chest covered the face, and interfered with breathing and access to the mouth. In his new design, the cap and jacket are made of strong linen, and the cap does not extend down the neck, but over the cheeks towards the chin to prevent it slipping backwards. On the top of the cap is a broad band to hold the wrist. The fixation of the arm is quite different from Tagliacozzi's. The arm is held in a linen cradle, which must fit perfectly, particularly round the elbow. From each side of this, nine bands run to the cap. But those who wish to operate exactly as he did should consult his book.[7] Benedict had the cap divided into several sections to make it easier to change the dressings, and to prevent chafing by the pus from the arm.[8]

As after every operation, the work of the surgeon is now only half-done, and he must show that he is a surgeon in the fullest sense of the word by his skilful after-care—particularly necessary in plastic oper-

---

[5] C. F. von Gräfe, Organischer Ersatz der Nase aus der Armhaut, *J. Chir. Augenheilk,* **22,** 8 (1834).

[6] [Tinct. benz. co.]

[7] See p. 14, n. 50.

[8] T. W. G. Benedict, *Beiträge zu den Erfahrungen über die Rhinoplastik nach der deutschen Methode,* Breslau, 1828.

ations.[9] Healing can be expected if the patient feels well, if all functions are normal, and his pulse is quiet. If inflammation sets in, spreading from the flap to the arm and over the nose, the full antiphlogistic regime is used—keeping the room cool, etc. Locally, all stimulants are avoided, zinc ointment is applied, and the cotton wool is removed. If the patient complains of severe pain in the arm and face, but the inflammation is relatively slight, gangrene is to be feared. In such cases Gräfe would not use cooling, because it might hasten the death of the flap.[10]

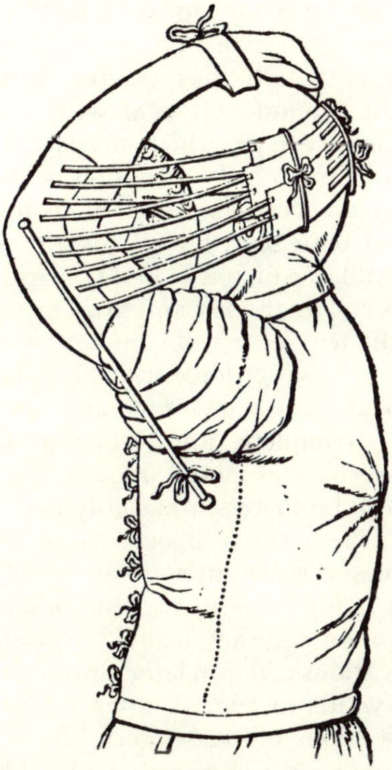

Fig. 5

In the Italian method, the flap is separated from the arm after 14–20 days. Gräfe was bold enough to separate it much earlier, as soon as union had taken place—even on the sixth day after its attachment. Fourteen days later, the columella is shaped and sutured at the same operation. This not only shortens the time, but the granulations on the inner surface of the nose and columella fuse to give the nose greater stability, and to keep it in a better shape. Also, the nourishment of the columella is ensured by its union with the lip. Before the nostrils are cut out, they must be carefully measured to leave enough skin to give prominence to the nose-tip. These measurements are made on the model, and transferred to the flap. The columella is inset, either into the lip or into the remnant of the old columella, with two interrupted sutures. Strips of lint, moistened with lead lotion, are placed in the nostrils, the wounds are dressed with zinc ointment, and the nose is wrapped in cotton wool. If union is satisfactory after several days, and the sutures are tending to cut in, they are removed, but the dressing is left for a few days longer.

[9] 'For who will praise a general who only knows how to face the enemy in open battle, and cannot also cope with their ambushes? Who will commend a sailor who can steer in a calm sea, but allows his ship to sink in a storm because of his inexperience?' Tagliacozzi, *de curtorum*, Vol. 2, Chapter 6, p. 20.

[10] Gräfe, *Rhinoplastik*, p.148.

Gräfe's concern is then to maintain the vitality of the new nose, protecting it from cold with cotton wool, and exposing it to the sun. He uses little lead tubes in the nostrils, as recommended by Tagliacozzi, to prevent them contracting, and he lifts the nose-tip with an instrument that he invented, the *eductor*, reinforced by external compression. The details of these are omitted here, as all such devices are useless. Living tissues, with the exception of bone, never retain the effects of even long-continued pressure, and it is the same with Gräfe's *compressorium* as with Tagliacozzi's *tectorium*. Transplanted skin tends to contract symmetrically, and there is nothing to stop this if it is not kept stretched by the underlying tissues. Skin has this tendency to such a degree that an incision, without loss of tissue, will gape. Although this retraction will be reversed without treatment, and the wound will heal with no residual contracture, this never happens in a flap, which needs the greatest care to get it to heal without bunching up. Contraction is all the more likely if it lies free and unsupported over a cavity, such as the nose. Its under-surface becomes covered with scar, which contracts more than the epidermal surface, so that a flap which is at first lax, and moves with every breath, becomes convex. The thicker and firmer the skin, and the larger the flap, the more the new nose will come to look like a real one, but this will never happen, however long or firmly it is held with instruments.[11] Even if the apparatus is worn for several years, until long after the scarring process is complete, and, when it is removed, the nose retains for a time the shape imposed upon it, the skin's innate tendency to contract will still be there—it has only been artificially delayed. This is one of the drawbacks of plastic surgery: even if a good appearance has lasted for several months, contraction will then destroy much of its beauty. It is the same with many other operations: the patient, after an operation for cataract, leaves hospital delighted that he can see, but the complications come on later, and they are often not recorded, because no one wants to review patients who have gone blind again. But the complications of eye surgery are no reason to abandon such worthwhile operations; rather they should spur the surgeon to develop less traumatic techniques and more effective after-care. It is the same with the contraction of the skin that sometimes, but not always, spoils plastic operations. Artificial devices are no use here. Man cannot change the laws of nature. Operations will only be successful if they are based on a knowledge of physiological and pathological processes.

[11] 'Thus the flap should not be the same length as the nose, but should be cut longer and wider from the arm.' Tagliacozzi, *de curtorum*, Vol. 2, Chapter 15, p. 56.

VON GRÄFE'S FIRST OPERATION BY THE GERMAN METHOD[12]

In 1817, Gräfe treated a woman aged 24, who had lost the tip of her nose from a phagedaenic ulcer that had started seven years before. The septum and alar cartilages had been destroyed, so that the nose was flat, and she could only breathe with great difficulty through a very small opening. The ulcer was healed in six weeks by sublimate internally and externally.[13] After waiting for six months to see that there was no recurrence, Gräfe began the operation on 11 September 1817 by opening up the nose and freshening the stump. A flap was raised on the arm, and sutured to the nose. When the harness was in place, the patient complained of pain in her elbow and shoulder. On the fourth day union was complete, and all the sutures were removed. The position of the arm was not causing the patient so much discomfort. The wound on the arm discharged pus freely. Beautiful granulations developed on the raw surface of the flap, and good thick pus was secreted. The flap was separated from the arm on the sixth day. A little blood oozed out of the cut end, and it became pale and cold, but recovered the next day. Its weight was supported by sticking-plaster, and it was kept warm with dressings. On the fourteenth day Gräfe shaped the columella, and set it into the lip. The flap had already become very thick, although not as much as in the Italian method. In October the *compressor* and the *eductor* were applied to lift the tip of the nose. The nostrils remained excoriated for a long time, and they had to be enlarged to relieve the tension of the *eductor*. A strong growth of hair on the new nose was singed off, and the redness of the scar, and the pallor of the flap, were treated by inunction of Hoffman's balsam.[14]

The disadvantages of Gräfe's method are even greater than the Italian, and so outweigh the reputed advantages that it is difficult to decide whether it should be used at all. It is difficult to dress the arm while it is attached to the head, without pulling on the flap. For the minimum of six days that the arm must be held to the head, the wound on the arm discharges pus, which irritates the skin, and upsets the patient by its smell. The problem of the weight of the ligature-rods, of which at least eight are needed, has already been mentioned;[15] these can, however, be replaced by simple interrupted sutures, as Gräfe himself has done. But a much greater hazard is that, when the flap has been detached from

---

12 Gräfe, *Rhinoplastik,* p. 174.

13 [Corrosive sublimate, mercuric chloride.]

14 [Alcoholic solution of balsam of Peru and essential oils.]

15 [See p. 40.]

the arm, it is only nourished through the newly formed scar. This was also true of Tagliacozzi's method, but there the flap was attached for longer, so that success was more certain. It might be said that, if the attachment is not to be trusted, then it should not be divided so soon; but this is getting back to Tagliacozzi. The Indian method is quite different: the pedicle of the flap can be left as long as necessary, without the least discomfort, until it is excised to remove the final disfigurement from the patient's face. The few complications, the minimal danger from the wound on the forehead, and the linear scar or small patch on the forehead are much less of a contraindication than the danger of the death of a flap which is raised on a distant part of the body. The Indian method is now used much more frequently for rhinoplasty than Tagliacozzi's and Gräfe's methods, which are more tedious, need more experience, and have the greater danger of failure. The patient, who should have rest and comfort after any operation, is so apprehensive of the cramped position with his arm fastened to his head that, if given the choice, he prefers the Indian method, and discounts the scar on his forehead. This position is certainly not held as long with Gräfe's method as with Tagliacozzi's, but the wound on the arm is fresh and painful. The arm swells, so that the bandage becomes too tight, and has to be changed, and it is difficult to apply anti-inflammatory treatment. Sometimes the arm is so swollen that it covers the whole face, and is pressed against it. Even though the arm is only up there for a short time, it can excoriate the face, and make eating and drinking impossible, which are difficult enough after Tagliacozzi's operation. It is easy to see all the dangers for the flap—only by good luck will it survive.

Apart from Gräfe, who used his method repeatedly,[16] Benedict has done it twice,[17] and Dybeck, in Warsaw, once (calling it Garranne's method), for an ala destroyed by syphilis.[18] Dieffenbach's modification is worth reporting as historically interesting, although the operation was a failure: he raised a flap on the upper arm, with a narrow pedicle, so that, when the elbow was fixed in front of the forehead, the flap came down from above, instead of coming up to the face from below. He thought that this would increase its blood-supply, and make the position of the arm more comfortable, Instead of a harness he used strips of

---

[16] C. F. von Gräfe, Neue Beiträge zur Kunst Theile des Angesichts organisch zu ersetzen, *J. Chir. Augenheilk.* **2,** 27 (1821).

[17] See n. 8 above.

[18] A. F. Dybeck, Glücklich ausgeführter Ersatz eines Nasenflügels, *J. Chir, Augenheilk.* **5,** 364 (1823).

sticking-plaster. On the sixth day the columella was gangrenous, and the whole flap gradually separated by the tenth day. It healed on the arm in 3–4 weeks, and, although markedly contracted, it was big enough to have allowed a second attempt.[19]

[19] Dieffenbach, *Erfahrungen*, Vol. 1, p. 33 (1829).

6
THE INDIAN METHOD

The method of rhinoplasty practised by the Indians has already been described.[1] To justify calling it the Indian method, it is not necessary to copy this rather crude technique exactly, as long as the principle is retained, and only the details are altered. Carpue, for example, noted that the nose made by the 'Artist of Poona' had no columella separating the nostrils.[2] But all noses made in Europe by the Indian method have nostrils and a columella. Others before Carpue had attempted this operation, but it had either failed or had not attracted much attention, so that he deserves the credit, by his successful operations and by his writings, for introducing the Indian method to Europe. With as much right as Gräfe, who called his modified Italian method the 'German' method, Carpue could have made himself out to be the inventor of an 'English' method, but this never crossed his mind.

The Indian method uses the skin of the forehead or other neighbouring parts, in contrast to the Italian method, where the flap is brought from a distance, either from the upper arm, the forearm, or the hand. Tagliacozzi used local skin to reconstruct the ear, without any knowledge of the Indian method, but he never made a nose out of the forehead. These terms are now established by common usage, and they should be retained. The essentials of the Indian method for all plastic operations, not only rhinoplasty, are: preparation of the defect, raising a nearby flap on a narrow pedicle by which it remains attached, turning the flap into the defect without tension, and suturing it into place. It is known that, in India, lips and ears, as well as noses, are reconstructed. The 'Artist', who was summoned to Poona to treat Cowasjee, offered to 'operate on the eldest son of the British native-ambassador at the Paishwah's court, who had lost part of his upper lip, but who, it appears, did not submit to the experiment'.[3] Rhinoplasty is now, as it always was, the most common plastic operation, and it serves to represent them all. Many of the observations made about it will also apply to the reconstruction of other parts. The term 'Indian' can,

---

[1] See p. 12.

[2] Carpue, *Two successful operations*, p. 40.

[3] Ibid. p. 102.

therefore, be used for operations that do not originate in India, but are based on the principle of reconstruction with skin from near the defect.

It is much easier to do an operation if you have seen it carried out by others, rather than simply hearing it described. The technique can be practised on the cadaver, but the competence that comes from knowledge of the physiological and pathological processes will always be lacking. The information that Carpue had received about the Indian method was very incomplete, and it is therefore interesting for us to study the details of his first case.

CARPUE'S FIRST OPERATION BY THE INDIAN METHOD[4]

In the month of September, 1814, I was applied to by an Officer in his Majesty's army, whose nose was in a mutilated state . . . I had long wished for an opportunity of performing the operation; and, for the space of fifteen years, had constantly recommended it to my pupils. The patient went to Egypt in the year 1801; but, becoming affected with a liver complaint, was obliged to return to Europe. At Malta, as well as previously in Egypt, mercury, the usual remedy in such a case, was employed . . . he went to Ireland, where the same plan was pursued . . . The consequence of this excessive use of mercury was, that the septum of the nose began to slough . . . the mercury was at length laid aside . . . he gradually recovered his health; but with the loss of the septum, all the anterior part of the cartilage, and, in truth, the whole front of the nose, a small portion of the alae, or sides of the nostrils, excepted. The nasal bones remained entire.

[But] the constitution had been impaired by the liver complaint and its improper treatment. The question to be decided was, is this a fair case for trial? I wished to determine that point; and, therefore, under pretext of preparing for the operation, I made incisions near the remains of the alae. The wounds healed . . . I next formed a nose of wax, and commenced a series of experiments on the dead subject . . . . At length, on the 23rd of October . . . I proceeded to perform the operation. The patient's forehead was unusually low, and, on that account, some days previously to performing the operation, I removed the hair, by the roots, from the scalp; the integuments of that part being required to form the septum or base of the nose . . . my fear being, that the hair would grow, and prevent adhesion. Having well ascertained the size of the graft required, by means of a wax model, which I then flattened, and laid on the forehead, I drew the outline round it with red paint. This done, the patient leaped upon a table, with his head supported by a pillow, refused to be held. Nor did he make the smallest complaint during the operation.

---

[4] Ibid, pp. 81ff [taken from Carpue (1816), rather than re-translate the German version].

I now made an incision on the right, and then on the left; and dissected out a sufficient quantity of the face . . . to receive what was to be dissected from the forehead. I made a simple incision for receiving the septum . . . I began that part of the operation which belongs to the forehead, by making an incision along the lines I had drawn. I then dissected the integuments, merely leaving the pericranium. The angular artery, on the left side, bled freely; but the loss of blood was very inconsiderable, and there was no occasion for tying the artery. The part which was dissected, and which hung down, became of a purple colour; and the patient, at this period, informed me, that his forehead felt extremely cold. I applied warm sponges, which afforded great relief.

My next steps were to make the *turn* of the dissected parts, and, introduced the septum into the incision of the upper lip, where I confined it by ligature. After this, I brought the integuments exactly into contact with the integuments on the left side, and fixed them also by two ligatures; and, then I did the same on the right. I introduced lint to distend the nostrils, and applied straps of adhesive plaster to keep the integuments in contact . . . my concluding care was to bring the edges of the integuments on the forehead, and between the eyebrows, as near together as possible, and keep them so by means of adhesive plaster.

A brother officer of the patient having been in the room during the operation, and kept an account of the time by his watch, I am enabled to state that it occupied exactly a quarter of an hour; the dissection having employed nine minutes, and the ligatures six. After this, the application of the necessary bandages, changing the linen of the patient, sponging away the blood, and placing the patient in bed, consumed twenty-two minutes more; making in the whole thirty-seven minutes. Short, however, as was the time, had it not been for my habit of frequently performing operations on English soldiers, I must have been astonished at the fortitude with which my patient went through this. When it was past, he observed, that, 'It was no child's play—extremely painful—but there was no use in complaining . . . . .' His resolution is the more worthy of observation, because there was, in his case, no prior example of success, either in my own practice, or in England, to support his confidence in me, or mine in the certainty of the result.

In the night, there was haemorrhage, but not in any quantity. On the third day, I took off the dressings . . . and I had the high satisfaction to hear the officer, before alluded to, exclaim, from the foot of the bed, 'My G-d, there *is* a nose!' . . . . The parts adhered . . . the nose was of the same colour with the face. Meantime, it was perfectly flat, and rose and fell with every inspiration and expiration . . . . The flatness of the nose alarmed me . . . and, to remedy this, I thought of procuring the air-bladder of a fish, which I proposed to introduce into the nose, and then inflate, with the design of raising the point of the nose. My apprehensions, however, on this, as in other parts of the cure, were groundless. Nature worked with me, and raised the nose by her own means.

Fourth day. Cut away two ligatures, and dressed the forehead, which appeared in a very healthy state . . . . *Sixth day.* All the ligatures removed . . . . *Ninth day.* Nose became oedematous . . . . Within a month afterward, the nose began to decrease in size.

Four months after the operation, I made a dissection of the integuments on the bridge of the nose, which I united from the turn, which had disappeared, and confined them by ligature; being of opinion, that if, in this cold climate, I followed that part of the Indian method, which consists in removing the turn, by which is carried on the circulation from the parent parts, the nose would slough . . . .In no other particular of importance, have I departed from the Indian method. The oedema at length subsided, but left the nose very flat. Subsequently, however, granulations formed, and the nose experienced a healthy enlargement . . . . I caused the patient to place himself in such a situation as allowed his profile to be drawn upon a wall; and, by making the comparison every two or three days, I had the pleasure to see its gradual increase demonstrated. In the present state of the nose, though there is neither bony or cartilaginous septum, yet the anterior or projecting part is solid, and has every appearance of a natural nose. The nostrils are gradually growing bigger,[5] and the secretion takes place as usual. The forehead was healed in three months . . .

In January 1815, Carpue carried out a second rhinoplasty in exactly the same way, except that the right side of the flap was attached to a part of the ala that remained, and the new columella was attached to the stump of the old one. Healing was complete in 10 days.[6]

VON GRÄFE'S FIRST INDIAN RHINOPLASTY

Gräfe, in 1817, was the first to follow Carpue with the Indian method. He advised that any large prominence on the stump of the nose should be removed at a preliminary operation, and rhinoplasty carried out only when this had completely healed. But there is no reason why the removal of these projections cannot immediately precede the rhinoplasty. He seems to be making the whole procedure unnecessarily complicated, and subjecting the patient to twice the amount of pain. I do not know whether he has changed his technique as a result of experience over the past 20 years. He also recommended preparing the stump by parallel incisions, and removing the intervening strip. But, when parts of the nose can still be used, simple excision of the margins

5 [Zeis] It is hard to understand how nostrils can grow bigger on their own—this must be an illusion. I have only ever seen them contract.

6 Carpue, *Two successful operations*, pp. 91ff.

is enough to provide contact for the flap. His groove-forming incisions should, in any case only be made on the sides of the nose, without carrying them over the bridge, for this is where the pedicle will lie, and the flap cannot be sutured there. Gräfe carried the pedicle over intact skin, without setting it in. He inserted the sutures in the defect before the flap was raised, so that it could be sutured into place more quickly. Recent experience is against this, for the reunion of completely separated parts has shown that there is no danger if completely or, as here, nearly completely separated parts are not immediately reattached; there is even an advantage in waiting until bleeding has stopped, and the serous stage has been reached.

Case report In July 1817, Gräfe operated on a woman aged 51, with a cancer of the nose that had started as an ulcer 18 years before. This had been cured in eight weeks by internal medication, and sublimate externally, leaving her with the loss of nearly the whole of the cartilaginous part of her nose, and the scar of the ulcer on her cheek. Gräfe waited two months, to see that there was no recurrence, before raising the forehead flap. The operation followed his principles (as above). The next day the flap was red and swollen, but the edges of the wound secreted coagulating lymph, which held them together. The sutures were removed on the third and fourth days, and the pedicle was divided three weeks later.

Gräfe felt that the Indian method should only be used when other methods were impracticable, and that the skin of the forehead should be freely mobile, neither too thick nor too thin, and the forehead not too low.[7] But the skin can never be too thick for transplantation, and it is best when covered with sebaceous follicles. With regard to a low forehead—this did not prevent Carpue using hairy skin after it had been shaved. Regrowth of hair is treated by plucking (singeing is no good), and, when this has been done once, the growth of hair on the flap stops completely. Gräfe also recommends the Indian method when the bridge of the nose has been destroyed. The pedicle of a forehead flap is the best way of reconstructing this area, for the Italian and German methods can only restore the lower part of the nose. He also regards a predisposition of the patient to erysipelas as a contraindication to the

[7] C. F. von Gräfe, Fall von Rhinoplastik aus der Stirn, *J. Chir Augenheilk.* **12.** 11, (1828).

Indian operation, but this must also apply to the other methods, as he himself experienced in one of his modified Italian operations.[8]

Gräfe, whose outstanding contributions to so many aspects of surgery will always be recognized, is now noted for his preoccupation with complicated instruments; this is at a time when the general policy is to keep things as simple as possible. Surgery will not be advanced by the invention of new instruments, which are expensive, and which need special training in their use. They are also difficult to make, so that the surgeon is dependent on the instrument-maker, if he is not to be let down by faulty instruments during an operation. Time has shown whether Gräfe was right to say that the Indian method was the preliminary experiment, and that the Italian is the completed work of art.[9] It is 20° years since *chirurgia curtorum* was revived. Since then, many plastic operations, the majority with very satisfactory results, have been carried out in Germany, England, and France. New techniques have been developed, not only for rhinoplasty, but also for the reconstruction of other parts. Now it may be asked: which method is superior—reconstruction with neighbouring skin, or with skin from a distance? Undoubtedly the former!

The disadvantages of the Italian operation are the danger of failure, the great hardship for the patient, and the dissimilarity of the skin of the arm and the face; these outweigh the fear of an unsightly scar on the forehead and the danger of exposing the skull. The number of Indian operations now far exceeds the Italian. In special cases, where the Indian method is contraindicated, the Italian is still needed, so that it will not disappear again. But many of the things that Gräfe held against the Indian operation are not regarded as important by modern surgeons, who have been getting very satisfactory results, and saving the patients from the tortures of the Italian, and even the Gräfe, operation.

THE INDIAN OPERATION AFTER CARPUE AND GRÄFE

In England, where the art that was transplanted from India to Europe first took root, the operation has not often been carried out. Even Carpue does not seem to have gone any further; at least, no later plastic operations by him are known. Hutchison did a rhinoplasty in 1818 for a woman who had lost her nose from gangrene following erysipelas, and who could not earn her living because of her hideous deformity; the

[8] See p. 40, n. 5.

[9] Gräfe, *Rhinoplastik*, p. 65.

nose was satisfactory, but the nostrils contracted.[10] In 1823, in London, Davies operated on a man who had lost his nose and upper lip from syphilis; the nostrils contracted because the patient did not keep them packed with lint for long enough.[11] No other plastic operations in England are known,[12] although Syme has recently carried out some small procedure.[13]

In Germany, Gräfe was followed by von Walther,[14] Chelius,[15] Textor,[16] Bünger,[17] Blasius,[18] Heidenreich,[19] and Ruppius.[20] In Russia, Höfft did an Indian rhinoplasty in 1823.[21]

In France plastic surgery had a difficult start. Even in 1819 Percy could write that so much pain was too high a price to pay for a very imperfect nose, and that it was better to have one made of wood or leather, which could be attached to spectacles.[22] Thomain, in 1825, seems to have been the first to have done a forehead rhinoplasty.[23]

---

[10] A. C. Hutchison, Case in which the nasal operation has been recently performed, *Edinb. med. surg. J.* **14**, 344 (1818).

[11] J. Davies, A case where the Taliacotian operation was successfully performed, *Lond. med. Repos.* **21** 39 (1824)

[12] [But see p. xiii n. 11.]

[13] J. Syme, Praeternatural aperture in the nose. Closure by transplanting a flap of skin, *Edinb. med. surg, J.* **44**, 5 (1835). [James Syme (1799–1870), professor of clinical surgery in Edinburgh (1833), had already done a rhinoplasty (see *Lancet* **2**, 613 (1834–35), although later he came to prefer a prosthesis.]

[14] See p. 79, n. 22.

[15] M. J. Chelius, *Handbuch der Chirurgie,* Vol. 2, Heidelberg, p. 546 (1834).

[16] K. Textor, Rhinoplastik aus der Stirnhaut nach der indischen Methode, *J. Chir. Augenheilk.* **6,** 374 (1824).

[17] See p. 21 n. 20.

[18] E. Blasius, *Handbuch der Akiurgie,* Halle (1831).

[19] F. W. Heidenreich, Heilung eines Krebses an der Nase mit vollständiger Herstellung der Gestalt und Farbe. *J. Chir. Augenheilk,* **20,** 456 (1833).

[20] J. K. Ruppius, Eine Rhinoplastik aus der Stirnhaut *Z. ges. med.* **4,** 243 (1837)

[21] S. F. Höfft, Rhinoplastices Britannicae seu Nasi restituti ope insiti a fronte ademti corii specimen, *Commentationes soc. phys.-med. apud univ. liter. Caes. Mosquensem instit.* **3,** 33 (1823)

[22] P.-F. Percy and C. Laurent, *Dictionaire des sciences médicales* Vol. 36, Paris, p. 74 (1819).

[23] [See p. 16, n. 65]

7

THE INDICATIONS FOR PLASTIC SURGERY

THE GENERAL INDICATIONS

The following general observations are made to demonstrate the importance of plastic surgery. The indications for each operation are given in the individual chapters.

Loss of the nose

Rhinoplasty in India owes its origin to the custom of punishing thieves, deserters, and, particularly, adulterers by cutting off their noses and ears, which was practised in olden times, and is still practised today. It is no wonder that the art of making noses developed much later in Europe, where such a grisly custom did not exist, and other causes of the deformity were relatively rare. In Europe the incentive was the frequent destruction of the nose by syphilis. Now that the technique is understood, it is also used for noses that have been lost from injury or operation. At present, when there are no wars, and duellists are generally less violent, it is not common for people to lose their noses from wounds, and most of the destruction needing plastic surgery is due to syphilis, or scrofulous and herpetic ulcers.[1] The latter are more common, since careful and regular treatment will prevent syphilis going on to destruction of the nose. If this does happen, either the patient is to blame for changing doctors, and not following instructions, or ignorant doctors have misused mercury, But the refusal of some doctors to prescribe mercury must also bear the blame for many a collapsed nose. Some hospitals have banned mercury. The patients leave them temporarily healed, but then the disease gradually breaks out again, without further infection. The hospital doctors never hear of this,

[1] [The term 'herpes' was used to cover a variety of diseases of the skin, of which the commonest were lupus, syphilis, and rodent ulcer. *Herpes exedens* was probably lupus, with some varieties of syphilis. *Herpes rodens* was probably rodent ulcer, with some lupus.]

because the patients, frightened of the harsh regime in the hospital, never go back there. Dupuytren was quite right:

> . . . recently venereal diseases have been treated solely by anti-inflammatory measures. But this fails to recognize that there are two elements in these diseases—the inflammatory and the syphilitic. Certainly the first symptoms of venereal disease are inflammatory, and should be treated as such. Sometimes this causes the symptoms to disappear, but it is a great mistake to assume that this has brought about a complete cure. Unless the syphilitic element has been destroyed, recurrence is always to be feared.[2]

Secondary syphilis appears as ulcers in the mouth, but it is not long before the nose becomes red, swollen, and painful, with a stinking discharge; it is usually too late to save it by anti-syphilitic treatment at this stage. The bone becomes necrotic, so that the nose collapses, giving a most unpleasant appearance in profile, although this is better from the front, as the skin is intact, and the tip of the nose is still present. This is the common picture, which can be seen on the streets every day. Less commonly, if the disease has not been treated, or only incompletely, the whole nose is destroyed, leaving a large hole. There may also be necrosis of the bones of the skull and orbit, with distortion of the eyelids, or ulcers in the mouth causing fusion of the cheeks to the jaws, which prevents the mouth opening. These complications make reconstruction of the nose more difficult. Sometimes other types of inflammation of the face, if not vigorously treated, produce similar, but less severe, effects on the nose.

The destruction caused by the herpetic and scrofulous ulcers of lupus is quite different.[3] The patients are young, with a scrofulous constitution, and the nose is affected after they have had scabby scalps, abscesses of glands, and joint disease as children. An ulcer with a thick scab on one nostril, or the nose-tip, resists all treatment, and penetrates deeply, destroying the nose. At puberty, for no apparent reason, the disease remits, and the ulcer heals. Sometimes herpes in adults will destroy other parts of the face, particularly the upper lip, as well as the nose. In contrast to syphilis, the bridge of the nose and the bony skeleton are mostly intact. Only the tip of the nose and the cartilage are missing, but this makes the appearance of the patient just as unsightly as with syphilis. Those who have lost their noses (called by the French '*rhinotmetes*') often have a network of scars on the face, which makes the

---

[2] G. Dupuytren, *Leçons orales de clinique chirurgicale, faites à l'Hôtel Dieu de Paris*, Vol. 1, Paris, p. 106 (1832).

[3] [See n. 1 above.]

operation more difficult; it is a bonus when the forehead is clear. The addition of a scar on the forehead is then hardly noticeable. Dieffenbach notes that rhinoplasty in patients with such scarring, particularly if the lips and mouth have been affected, often gives bad results. He has a wider experience of this condition than any other surgeon, and he states that previous scrofulous disease, even when the patient is in good health, is a much greater danger than *herpes exedens* or syphilis.[4]

But destruction by cancer is the most unsuitable of all for reconstruction. While any malignant ulceration remains, or any other underlying disease, there must be no reconstruction. Even if the area has healed, it is not worth putting the patient to the pain of a rhinoplasty, because it is impossible to be sure that the ulcer will not recur. Most of these patients are old, and they are not as concerned as the young about their appearance, so that they do not feel the need for this to be improved; in any case, they would only have a short time left to enjoy it. Further experience is needed to show whether Martinet de la Creuse was right to state that skin grafting after excision of cancer will prevent recurrence,[5] in which case, rhinoplasty would be indicated not only to improve the appearance, but even more for radical cure of the disease.

When the nose is missing, even the most beautiful face becomes a caricature. It can be improved by reconstruction, even though this bears only a distant resemblance to a normal nose. The eye is so used to seeing a nose on a human face, that even an ugly one is preferable to one that is partly or completely missing; there are many natural noses that do not conform to the artist's idea of beauty. The sufferings of someone who has lost his nose are made worse by the thought that he himself may be to blame. The layman makes no distinction, and even the innocent are subjected to insults, which make them go into hiding to avoid suspicion. Artificial noses of wood, silver, and other materials will disguise the deformity from a distance, but close to they make it worse—like a waxwork.

But the nose is not only for decoration—it is an important part of the respiratory system, controlling the entry of air. If it is missing, the mucous membrane becomes dry and crusted, which prevents the passage of air until the crusts are expelled by forcible exhalation. Air then passes directly into the larynx. The sense of smell is reduced or absent because of lack of moisture, and the patient cannot sneeze. Smell is always regarded as the least important of the senses, but there is a close

[4] Dieffenbach, *Erfahrungen*, Vol. 3, p. 17 (1834).

[5] See p. 178, n. 1

connection with taste, and people who cannot smell lose more than is commonly thought. Unclear speech, blockage of the tear-ducts, deafness from disease of the Eustachian tubes, and a foul smell also result from loss of the nose. All this, with a hideous appearance, makes these people unfit for employment and social life. It is the happy task of rhinoplasty to relieve all these misfortunes.

Blindness is a great misfortune, but it may be worse to have no nose:

> . . . a blind man arouses pity, but a man without a nose, horror and loathing, and people are apt to regard the deformity as a just punishment for his sins. This division of diseases, or even more their consequences, into blameworthy and blameless is strange. The victim who has lost his nose finds no pity, least of all from the hypocrites who are always ready to say that it is all his own fault. As if people with noses were always guiltless! No one ever asks whether the nose was lost because a beam fell on it, or whether it was destroyed by scrofula or syphilis.[6]

Reconstruction of the mouth

This is most commonly needed for fusion of the lips to each other, or to the jaws, following the cure of syphilis with mercury. Anyone whose mouth has been reduced to a small hole suffers endless torment. He can only survive on fluids, and even if he can put solid food in his mouth he cannot chew it, because he cannot separate his jaws. Although the mouth is something negative—a hole—it is necessary to use reconstructive techniques that may truly be regarded as 'plastic', in order to make separation of the conjoined parts permanent.

Reconstruction of the lips

This is needed after noma, carcinoma, gangrene, or injury. The patient suffers severely, not only from his hideous appearance (like a ravening animal), but saliva and food dribble out of his mouth, and his whole nutrition deteriorates. His teeth, in contact with the air, become black and brittle. His gums thicken and harden, like mucous membrane that has been transplanted on to the surface of the body. His tongue protrudes through the gaps in his teeth, and his speech becomes unintelligible.[7]

---

[6] Dieffenbach, *Erfahrungen*, Vol. 3, p. 39 (1834).

[7] 'Is it so small a feat, then, to remove such vile ruination? That the face should attain its former beauty? That you who have been like a monster, a source of curiosity, should presently appear more like a human being? Reflect how close at hand is hope, how much more certain than prayer, and how short is your present suffering.' Tagliacozzi, *de curtorum*, Vol. 2, Chapter 14, p. 50.

Destruction of the soft palate

Here the difficulties of repair are so great that there is little chance of success. Dieffenbach has attempted it, but no one else seems to have copied him.[8]

The loss of one or both eyelids

This may lead to blindness. The whole lid need not be missing for this to happen: severe ectropion, lagophthalmos,[9] or scar contracture pulling the lid away from the eye leave the conjunctiva exposed. The eye, unprotected from air and light, becomes grossly inflamed, the conjunctiva thickens, the cornea becomes opaque, and the patient goes blind. Operations to restore the eyelids certainly count as plastic surgery. But there is no need to include here those that are dealt with in every text-book of ophthalmology. The term 'blepharoplasty' should only be used for reconstruction for actual loss of tissue.

Loss of the ear

This is less important. The deformity can be covered by the hair, and there is no effect on hearing. The operation to create a free-standing structure, such as an ear, is extremely difficult; at first, the transplanted skin may look like an ear, but in the end it always crumples up. The term 'otoplasty' should only be used for the restoration of parts of the ear—the upper half or the lobe.

Fistula of the trachea

This causes loss of the voice. A chronic fistula can be cured by transplantation (bronchoplasty).

Reconstruction of the foreskin (posthioplasty)

A man who would submit to having a new foreskin made must be as vain as one who wishes to have his ear reconstructed. It is so unimportant a part, and so easy to get used to its loss, that there are never urgent indications for operation. However, it appears that Jews, who had been baptized, sometimes wished to have new foreskins made; for this reason

[8] See p. 171.

[9] [Inability to close the eye, without eversion of the eyelid.]

they were known as *recutiti*.[10] Illogically, the operation to cure adhesion of the foreskin to the glans is also called 'posthioplasty'.

Fistulae in the male urethra

Operations to close these are much more important. In the perineum, they commonly follow extravasation of urine from the false passage of rough catheterization. In the distal part of the penis they are usually due to syphilitic ulceration, but sometimes to wounds, or other causes. The inability to pass water in a straight stream means that, unless the patient gets undressed, he wets his clothes. But at least he can hold his water, which is not the case with a vesico-vaginal fistula.

Vesico-vaginal fistula

The sufferings of a woman with the involuntary and continuous dribbling of urine from a vesico-vaginal fistula are so great that Dieffenbach deserves the deepest gratitude of the patients, and of the doctors who have to look after them, for his discovery of new and successful operations. It is hard for a man to use a urine bag, but even harder for a woman, where the urine runs past and into her shoes. The urine makes her thighs raw, she always smells of urine, and no one will stay near her; to keep herself clean is an expense that a poor woman cannot afford. Difficult childbirth, and poor care during it, is the commonest cause. Often there is not just a split, but pieces of the vagina and posterior wall of the bladder are torn out. The damage would not be so great if the torn, but still attached, tissues were at once sutured. After a time, the flaps become scarred and contracted, and it is very difficult to open them out, and to get them to heal to the margins of the fistula. Fistulae are less commonly due to syphilis; these are smaller than after childbirth—often so small that they are hard to find, and can only be seen by injecting the bladder with coloured fluid. But the disability is the same as with a large opening, and the cure is nearly as difficult. It is easier to reduce the size of a large fistula than to close it completely, because of the continuous seepage of urine.

Reconstruction of the scrotum (oscheoplasty)

This is needed after lacerations. In many cases, the testicles are exposed because the lacerated skin has retracted. All that is needed is to

---

[10] See p. 182, no. 4.

bring the skin together over the testicles; but this is easier said than done, because scrotal skin heals badly. Sometimes the skin has been destroyed by gangrene, or it is so diseased that it must be excised. Even in a grossly diseased scrotum, as in elephantiasis, the testicles may remain healthy. The surgeon must then preserve them, and advance local skin from the belly or inner sides of the thighs to cover them. The few cases in which this operation has been carried out have been relatively successful.

Tenotomy

The cure of feet and other joints deformed by contracted tendons, by dividing the tendons and stretching the fibrous tissue that forms as they heal, bears some relation to a plastic operation. I feel, therefore, that it is necessary to devote some space to it, without deviating too far from my purpose. The creation of fibrous tissue in the gap is the work of nature, but the art consists of stretching the newly forming tissue, without which there would be no benefit. Recent work has enabled tendons to be divided without danger. At first, this was only applied to the division of the Achilles tendon for congenital club-foot, but now it can be used for all tendon contractures.

RELIEF OF DISABILITY

It can be seen that it is not only vanity that makes patients undergo plastic operations. Even if these operations are not life saving, they are not simply to improve appearance; they are of the greatest value in relieving disability. In many cases, when a patient needs a surgical operation anyway, it is possible, by a small addition, to turn it into a plastic operation; this promotes healing, so that the patient recovers more quickly. The extra pain is of no account in relation to the benefit received. The excision of the lower lip for cancer, for example, leaves the patient in a miserable state, if the wound cannot be closed. With a large defect, simple closure is not possible, but the lip can always be reconstructed by a skin flap. Even if such an artificial lip has no red margin and no muscle, the patient is still much better off than one whose teeth and jaw are exposed, with saliva dribbling out. Again, after amputation of the breast, there is no comparison between leaving the wound to heal by granulation, and covering it with a skin flap. The place from which the flap was taken must then, of course, suppurate and granulate, but this is of little importance, because of the advantage gained. The general rule used to be to pull the edges of the wound together as hard as possible, but the sutures were often under such tension that they cut out. However, there was no alternative, until plastic surgery was introduced by surgeons who were familiar with the use of flaps in other situations.

The criticism may be made of plastic surgery that a reconstructed nose or eyelid is less perfect than the normal. No one knows this better than the surgeon who has carried out plastic operations. But this should not damp his enthusiasm—rather it should inspire him. Twenty or so years ago, who would have imagined all that has since been accomplished? Is this work now finished, or is there hope of even greater improvement in the future?

THE AGE OF PATIENTS FOR PLASTIC OPERATIONS

The deformities that call for plastic surgery can occur at any age. But children are too delicate for most plastic operations, and their inability to co-operate makes it impossible to carry out operations that need the greatest courage and endurance on the part of the patient, such as repair of the soft palate. Since a reconstructed nose in a child will be too small in adult life, it is necessary to wait until his head is fully grown. The operation for hare-lip is indicated in childhood, but this can also be postponed.

In considering the upper age of patients for plastic surgery, it is cruel to put pressure on very old people, who may only have a little time to live after the operation. They have long been accustomed to their deformities, and have, in any case, withdrawn from the bustle of life, passing their days in solitude. Apart from this, the outcome of all plastic operations in old people is very uncertain. The poor vitality of their skin prevents the primary healing necessary for transplantation. But there are exceptions to this rule, and, even in the very old, transplantation may be carried out to reduce the disability after, for example, excision of carcinoma of the lip, or amputation of the breast.

Middle age and youth carry the best prognosis. These people still have the greater part of their lives before them, and they have the will to recover and to return to a normal life.

THE GENERAL CONDITION OF THE PATIENT

Emergency and life-saving operations must often be carried out without consideration for the constitution of the patient, his underlying diseases, or his age. But before any plastic operation, these must be attended to. Deformities due to injury are much less common than those due to disease, which is often not cured at the time that surgical help is required. The surgeon must take the greatest care, not just to have the assurance of other doctors who treated the patient earlier, but to decide for himself whether the syphilis is quiescent. The length of time since the ulcers were healed is often deceptive. These patients, after such an unhappy experience, should have become more careful. Unfortunately this is often not the case, and, although you might think that it would be difficult for people without noses to find an opportunity to become infected again, they seem to be able to manage it somehow.

The surgeon who wishes to carry out reconstructive operations must be very familiar with the treatment of syphilis, and must know how to differentiate syphilis from mercurial disease, which in many cases is very difficult. Sometimes there are only minor symptoms, disregarded by the patient, and no longer attributed to the earlier disease, which alert the surgeon: a small nodule, an indolent ulcer on the foot which resists all treatment, loss of hair, and so on. Even if one cannot be certain that gold is a reliable cure, it can give excellent results in cases where the presence of syphilis is not definitely established, and where one does not wish to use the full mercurial treatment; it will rapidly bring about a cure, and help to confirm the diagnosis. Deformity from syphilis only occurs in the severe forms of the disease, and, before carrying out a rhinoplasty on such a patient, it is sensible to give him Zittmann's[11] or Pollini's[12] decoction by mouth. One cannot be too careful about the cure of any underlying disease: syphilis, scrofula, herpes, lupus, cancer, and all the others that give rise to deformities needing plastic surgery. It is a great advantage if the surgeon, who will do the operation, has himself carried out the earlier treatment, for he will then be well placed to continue it after the operation. Whatever the underlying disease, it is always better if the operation is not carried out too soon after the cure has been completed.

In order to determine the healing power of the patient, a minor operation is usually carried out before the major one is undertaken. Often this is indicated on its own merits: a collapsed alar cartilage or nasal bridge can sometimes be freed and elevated for use in the rhinoplasty. If this tissue cannot be used, it is excised when the defect is prepared. If nothing of this sort is available, an incision is made in an unimportant site, and sewn up again, with no excuse other than: 'this has got to be done!'. This will show whether the patient's skin will heal

[11] [Sarsaparilla, calomel, and cinnabar—frequently used for syphilis.]

[12] [Sarsaparilla, cinchona, and antimonious sulphide.]

by first intention; if it does not, the patient should undergo general treatment, or should be sent into the country or to a spa.

Erysipelas is a frequent complication of plastic operations. Patients, who have never had it before, will not uncommonly develop it when a large piece of facial skin has been transplanted. It spreads over the head, to the back of the neck, or even over the whole of the back, with marked swelling and a high fever. Patients who have previously had erysipelas must be treated with particular care.

THE PROGNOSIS OF PLASTIC OPERATIONS

This is generally good, for, if the outlook is poor, the operation should obviously not be undertaken. But a 'knife-happy' surgeon can sometimes persuade an unsuitable patient to have an operation, only to run into complications. It is not so much of a disaster that the patient is not improved, and has only suffered in vain, but he may well be left in a worse state than before—as by the removal of tissue such as the remnants of his nose. He will be ill-served, after an unsuccessful rhinoplasty, by being sent away with a large hole in his face. This not only harms him, but harms the whole of plastic surgery, by frightening away other patients. Naturally, the prognosis varies with the cause of the original deformity: wounds with sharp weapons have the best prognosis, then syphilis, herpes, and, lastly, scrofula.

Many plastic operations are quite traumatic. A patient with a forehead rhinoplasty has a head wound, and all head wounds need very careful management. But the wound for a rhinoplasty is not made haphazardly, but according to a plan, with a sharp instrument; it does not injure the brain, the skull is not exposed, and the galea is preserved. The timing of the operation has been carefully chosen, so that there is no underlying illness that might lead to wound infection.

Most plastic operations are therefore successful, especially with careful after-treatment. There are reports of cases which were unsuccessful, or even fatal. But these were nearly all unconnected with the operation, and were related to chance illnesses, or underlying disease which was not detected.

THE REACTION OF THE PATIENT

This is of the greatest importance for the success of a plastic operation. In most cases it is favourable. Patients who have spent a long time in hiding, with no idea of the possibility of reconstruction, cheer up at once when they are told that they can be restored to a reasonable state.

They cannot wait for the operation, they have no anxiety about the pain, even when warned that it will be considerable, and they beg the surgeon to speed up the preparatory treatment. They have good reason for this, for they have nothing to lose by the operation. This is just the opposite of nearly all the other patients who need an operation to be cured of their disease, but who will thereby lose a part of their body—an arm, a leg, or a breast—and, in addition, may be looking forward gloomily to recurrence of a disease, which they may already have experienced once or more.

During the operation, the former group usually behave with great fortitude. They do not need to be restrained, and they do not groan, although the cutting of the skin, and injury to the many nerves of the face, undoubtedly cause severe pain, even in the most phlegmatic patients. After the operation they celebrate their cure, and do not go into hiding again.

Sometimes, however, the patient is depressed. This not only makes the surgeon's task more difficult, but, more serious, the depression of the spirits, as always, reduces the activity of the skin. There is then considerable danger that the flap will die. The prognosis for these patients must be unfavourable; they are not suitable for plastic operations, for their lack of spirit makes them more frightened of pain, which they genuinely feel more than those made of sterner stuff. In people with pale skin, fair hair, and blue eyes, a flap may very quickly become pale and cold, and there will be cramps and fainting during or after the operation. If the flap dies, this is due more to generally deficient nervous strength than to disordered blood-flow in the flap. However, this is not always the case, and sometimes even in these patients the results can be surprisingly good.

OTHER FACTORS TO BE CONSIDERED

Patients for plastic surgery come just as often from the upper classes as from the lower. Syphilis spares no one, rich or poor; all the other conditions needing plastic surgery occur equally in both classes. It is always best to operate in hospital, even with private patients. The patient will be better cared for, with doctors and good attendants to ensure that he will follow instructions; this is an important factor in the success of the operation. The wealthy patient can supply everything he needs (the poor man will only get this in a well-equipped hospital), but his independence makes him disobey instructions. If this spoils the result of the operation, the surgeon will get the blame.[13]

If a plastic operation is carried out privately it arouses the interest of the patient's friends. They come rushing round immediately after the operation to see the miracle, with no idea how it is done, expecting to find a nose like the Belvedere Apollo's.[14] Even if the patient has been told not to look in the mirror before he is allowed to, and all mirrors have been removed, the faces of his friends will soon tell him that his nose (that the surgeon said was so wonderful) is not up to their expectations. The surgeon knows that, for the first few days, it must look like a shapeless lump, if it is to be big enough to pass for a nose when all the swelling has gone down. He recognizes that redness and swelling of a flap are favourable signs, and he can be optimistic, because he can visualize what it will look like in the future. The patient may have been in a cheerful frame of mind, conducive to good healing. But then in come his inquisitive friends and neighbours who, even if they do not criticize the work of art, do not marvel at it, because naturally they know nothing about it. At his next visit, the surgeon finds the patient in tears, with this great pale blob sticking out of a red blotched face. The patient will not say what has happened, so as not to offend his surgeon. But he asks so many questions, that it is difficult to quieten him and then cheer him up. For this reason, all such visiting must be strictly forbidden from the start. The process of healing must be described to the relatives beforehand, so that they will be careful what they say.

Some patients ask, before the operation, how it is to be carried out, and, if they are intelligent, they can be told without frightening them. But there are others, without the slightest knowledge of physiology or pharmacology, who will not take any medicine that has been prescribed, until its action has been explained to them. They are simply trying to test their doctor (particularly if he is young), to see whether he knows his business, and is not just experimenting on them. Patients must be very well-educated to understand anything about medicine, and for most of them it is enough for the doctor to reply in general, noncommittal, and learned-sounding terms. But a doctor must be very

[13] 'Thus, let me issue a strong warning to surgeons, particularly as this art is new, in which, as in other parts of medicine, there is always the risk of receiving criticism as one's reward. For this is one of the misfortunes of doctors, that patients, however much they misbehave, not only do not blame themselves, but put all the blame on the doctors'. Tagliacozzi, *de curtorum*, Vol. 2, Chapter 2, p. 3.

[14] [Greek statue in the Vatican.]

sure of himself if he is to refuse to answer questions, without harming his reputation.

A surgeon will often be asked to give details of the operation, and he may demonstrate with the pattern of a rhinoplasty, for example, how this piece will form the columella, and that the ala. But he should also take this opportunity of reassuring the patient once again about the operation, being careful not to frighten him with anything that might sound dangerous.

8

THE PHYSIOLOGY AND PATHOLOGY OF SKIN FLAPS

TYPES OF SKIN

Some types of skin are unsuitable for transplantation. Even if a flap is left attached by a broad pedicle for a long time it must have a certain degree of vitality (which not every piece of skin possesses), if it is to survive. Tagliacozzi divided skin into four groups:

(1) the skin of the palm and sole, which is smooth and hairless, and cannot be lifted up in a fold;

(2) skin moved by a thin layer of muscle underneath it, e.g. the forehead;

(3) skin so closely interwoven with muscle that it could be called 'muscle-skin', e.g. the skin of the face;

(4) the skin over the rest of the body, which is sometimes hairy, but which does not move, and is easily separated from the underlying tissues.[1]

He regarded this last group as the only one suitable for transplantation, whereas we now prefer the forehead above all others.

By his method of reconstruction, using skin from a distance rather than near to the defect, Tagliacozzi had to choose a part that could be held close to the face for some time, so that he was limited to the upper arm or the forearm. For rhinoplasty, he recommended the former, because of the many tendons lying close under the skin of the forearm, and because the forearm is more often exposed, so that the scar is visible. The skin of the upper arm has the advantage of being thicker, but, as the Italian method prepares the flap before it is moved, there is no need to pay as much attention to the natural thickness of the skin as when a freshly raised flap is to be used. Apart from the underlying tendons, care must be taken not to raise a flap from a site where large

[1] Tagliacozzi, *de curtorum*, Vol. 2, Chapter 13, p. 38.

vessels and nerve trunks would be exposed. In Tagliacozzi's operation it was often impossible to avoid injuring the large veins in the arm. The bleeding was all the harder to stop because the flap was raised as a bridge; this made access to the vessels difficult, and the bleeding could only be controlled by pressure.

Tagliacozzi preferred the skin for transplantation to be mobile, but Blandin thinks that the more adherent the skin, as when there is no subcutaneous tissue, the greater the stability of the flap, and that it is even better when the underlying aponeurosis can be included.[2] Apparently he has never put this into practice, and, indeed, it should not be done. The galea must be preserved when a flap is raised on the forehead, because its removal exposes the frontal bone. As in other situations, the fibrous layer belongs to the underlying tissues, and not to the skin. The advantage of greater stability in the flap is offset by the inevitable sloughing of the fibrous layer.[3]

If a flap is left for some time before being attached, its nutrient vessels will enlarge, just as the collateral branches of an artery enlarge, when the main trunk is ligated, to carry the quantity of blood necessary to nourish the limb. The veins and lymphatics do the same, but more slowly, so that, if they are obstructed as well as the artery, the part remains oedematous for some time.

The thickness of the skin varies in different parts of the body, and there are even greater differences between individuals. The robustness of a person can usually be gauged by the thickness and texture of his skin, although too much reliance must not be placed on this. What is certain is that skin for transplantation can never be too thick. Thick skin contracts less, and the reconstructed part keeps its shape better. A thick flap is in less danger from disturbances of blood-supply, either inflow or outflow, and it heals better into its new bed because its edges provide a larger surface for adhesion. For these reasons the skin of the forehead is the best for transplantation, and this has now been established by repeated experience. The skin is best of all when it is covered with sebaceous follicles—not because it heals better, but because this is a sign of a particularly thick and vascular skin.

But the skin of the rest of the face has now been transplanted so often that there is no longer any doubt of its usefulness. However, its thinness and the presence of the eyes and the mouth prevent a large enough

---

[2] Blandin, *Autoplastie*, p. 97.

[3] [Here, and in several other places in the text, Zeis states that the galea aponeurotica is not to be included in a forehead flap. Other surgeons, however, made it clear that they raised the flap down to the pericranium—see p. 120.]

piece being taken to make a whole nose, and the resulting scar would put another deformity in the place of the original one. Thus, facial skin is unsuitable for rhinoplasty, which was Tagliacozzi's main concern, so that his opinion on this was correct. But there are many other smaller plastic procedures (repair of the ala, or the eyelid, or the closure of fistulae), for which it has often been used in recent times. Although the face is richly supplied with nerves, it can stand very severe injury without danger to life, and without causing nervous disorders.

Hairy scalp can also be used; either when the forehead is too low to provide enough skin for rhinoplasty, or the skin from behind the ear can be taken for otoplasty. The part of the scalp is shaved, and, when the hair regrows, it is plucked with eyebrow tweezers. It then stops growing, or becomes fine and silky, because the dissection of the flap takes place in the layer immediately under the skin, in which the hairs that penetrate the dermis have their roots. These roots become exposed, and they are not so well nourished as before. It is different with the fine hairs on the forehead or on the rest of the body, which do not penetrate so deeply. Their roots are in the dermis itself, so that they are included within the flap; they do not fall out, but grow more strongly than before, and appear closer together because of the contraction of the flap. If they spoil the appearance there is nothing to do but pluck them, but this is tedious as they slip out of the tweezers.

CONTRACTION OF THE FLAP

Every flap contracts by a quarter or a third in all dimensions immediately it has been raised, as Tagliacozzi knew very well.[4] This initial contraction, by which it naturally becomes thicker, is like the gaping of a skin wound—simply an example of the elasticity and contractility of the skin. But the process is not yet complete, and the skin will continue to contract for some time. If a flap is not immediately attached, it will tend to become spherical. It can only be held stretched out by the part to which it is sutured. Gräfe had an example of this in a flap from the arm, where the attachment was delayed too long.[5] But this can be seen in every rhinoplasty, where the columella, which is at first quite flat, contracts so much that it becomes a rounded bridge between the tip of

---

[4] 'People who have closely watched this sort of surgery have often seen the skin, after the second incision, gradually contract by some secret force, sometimes diminishing by an eighth, sometimes by a sixth, and on occasion even by a quarter, and losing as much in its width as in its length.' Tagliacozzi, *de curtorum,* Vol. 1, Chapter 15.

[5] Gräfe, *Rhinoplastik,* Pl. 4, Fig. 3.

the nose and the upper lip. Its raw surface naturally tends to scar and contract, so that the edges come together posteriorly, looking as though they had been sutured. The same happens to the free borders of the nostrils, which can thus easily become too small if they have not been made much too large in the first place.[6]

SEPARATION OF THE EPIDERMIS

This has sometimes been reported in a transplanted flap, although I have never seen it. It is more common after the reunion of a completely separated part. In one case of von Ammon's, the desquamation was preceded by a peculiar oedema, from lymphatic exudation under the epidermis, which appeared several days after the operation. Examination with the loupe showed that the new epidermis was different from the old, and more like that of the surrounding skin.[7]

TEMPERATURE CHANGES

The temperature of a completely separated piece of skin quickly comes to equal that of the surrounding air, as can be seen in any amputated part; the smaller the piece the quicker it cools. A skin flap nearly always becomes cooler as soon as it has been raised, and this is more marked the paler it is, the smaller its blood-supply, and the narrower its pedicle. If the cooling is not too severe, there is no need for anxiety about the survival of the flap, for in most cases the temperature rises as soon as it has been attached, without external warming. In winter, peripheral parts of the body become white and stiff from lack of blood, but, with careful warming, the circulation returns without ill effects; a flap is not subjected to such a degree of cold, as the temperature of the operating room is never so low. In most cases the cooling of the flap is slight, and its temperature only differs by a few degrees from the rest of the skin. After a few hours it has returned to normal, even when cold compresses are used to prevent inflammation in the recipient area; by the next day it is often higher than the surrounding skin.

---

[6] 'Therefore I enjoin doctors to follow this rule scrupulously, both because it is perfectly simple to cut too large a piece, while it is impossible later to make up for a deficiency, and so that they may not repent of their actions, and the dignity of their art.' Tagliacozzi, *de curtorum,* Vol. 2, Chapter 16. p. 59.

[7] F. A. von Ammon, Morioplastik, *Magazin ges. Heilk.* **39,** 173 (1837).

COLOUR CHANGES

At the same time as the fall in temperature the flap becomes paler, but this change is usually slight. After it has been sutured into place, its colour may hardly differ from the surrounding skin—particularly if it has a broad pedicle with large vessels in it, and if it has been undermined so that there is no tension when it is rotated, and, most important of all, if the skin is thick and healthy, without scarring. Even if the flap is pale at first, it recovers very quickly, and changes to red in the next few days. Sometimes it is terrifyingly white, but it still recovers quickly; there is no known case of a flap that has been lost immediately after it has been raised. All the disasters occur after several days, when the flap, which has been hot and congested, becomes insensitive, blue, cold, and then gangrenous. This is less common with the Indian method, where the pedicle can be left for a long time, than with the Italian and German methods, where the flap, after separation from the arm, is nourished entirely through the suture line. Gräfe had this experience in the case of a young man who had lost his upper lip and part of the cheek from typhus; the tissues round the defect were hard and fixed. Gräfe chose the Italian method, leaving the flap on the arm for more than two months. The attachment to the lip was carried out by Hedenus, his assistant at that time (1820). By the seventh day the flap was completely adherent, and it was separated from the arm. It was pale at first, but soon recovered. On the third day a leaden spot appeared on the left side, which spread until the whole transplant became gangrenous.[8] It seems that the rigidity of the tissues, to which the flap was sutured, was responsible for this unfortunate result.

CONGESTION IN THE FLAP

In many cases the flap goes blue a few hours after the operation, which indicates that the blood is stagnant. When this first happened in a rhinoplasty of Dieffenbach's, instead of worrying about gangrene, and using stimulants, he let blood out of the flap. He believed that the change of colour from red to blue meant that more blood was going into the flap than could get out, and he therefore thought it sensible to encourage the flap to bleed. He removed a swab that had been applied to control the bleeding, and immediately an artery started spurting briskly. This blood-letting worked well, for the flap quickly recovered

[8] Gräfe, Neue Beiträge p. 10 (1821).

its redness, and then became paler, and its temperature fell considerably.[9]

If it is not possible, as in this case, to encourage the edges of the flap to bleed, leeches on the flap or scarification are effective; cold compresses on the flap, the face, and the forehead will reduce the inflow of blood. It is much more common for a flap to be in danger from too much blood than from too little, but it is the discrepancy between reduced outflow and increased inflow that causes congestion.

In all his later cases, Dieffenbach used powerful general and local anti-inflammatory treatment for this circulatory problem, with very good results. Both von Ammon and I have confirmed the benefit of this regime. In France the cooling of transplanted flaps is also used, although Blandin does not agree that, when there is congestion, the inflow of blood must be reduced. While Dieffenbach advises the division of a large vessel in the pedicle, Blandin recommends that the pedicle should be designed to include a large artery. But this is impossible to determine in advance, and the surgeon cannot knowingly plan a flap with an artery in it; in any case, this is not desirable. Further experience will, in time, lead the French surgeons to the same conclusion that the Germans have already reached from their much greater experience.

HEALING BY FIRST INTENTION

All plastic operations depend on healing by first intention. To achieve this, the surgeon must exercise the greatest care before, during, and after the operation. Before undertaking any major plastic operation, particularly if its failure would leave the patient worse off than before, it must be established that there is no underlying disease. It is not enough to know that the patient is free of syphilis, for it is just as bad if he is still suffering from the effects of treatment with mercury. Delpech and Thomain both had the unhappy experience of fresh syphilitic ulcers developing after rhinoplastic operations in patients who had not been completely cured.[10] Often there is no definite disease, but simply a predisposition to infection, so that small cuts or pricks turn into chronic septic ulcers. Careful pre-operative treatment, and testing the patient's powers of healing, can prevent a poor result, but it is equally important to carry out the operation with all the precautions described in the

[9] Dieffenbach, *Erfahrungen,* Vol. 2, p. 72. (1830).

[10] Labat, *De la rhinoplastie,* p. 134 (1834).

operative sections of this book. Briefly, the most important measures to achieve primary healing are:

(1) to make the incision cleanly and vertically through the skin;

(2) to control the bleeding and to wait for the *stadium serosum* before suturing, i.e. until there is no more blood, but only watery fluid, coming out of the wound;

(3) to ensure that the wound edges are exactly apposed, without gaps, and, for this, twisted sutures are better than interrupted sutures, ligature-rods, or sticking-plaster.

The after-care is also very important. It is not enough to prescribe cold compresses—the patient and his relatives must be shown how to make these, for they are usually too small, and not changed often enough. The patient himself will often demand them, for he soon finds that they soothe the tension and heat in the wound on his forehead. The pressure of the twisted sutures may make the edges of the wound pale and bloodless for some time. If the thread is twisted too tightly round the needles, this can be harmful, but if it is done correctly it will encourage primary healing. If interrupted sutures have to be used, the wound edges much more often become red. A small degree of reddening does not matter, as the free use of cooling will control this slight inflammation. But when it is more marked, and, not only the wound edges, but the skin of the face and the donor site are inflamed, and the flap is bright-red, tense, and hot, local blood-letting is urgently needed to prevent the formation of pus. One must then just salvage as much as possible, and accept that primary healing, in all its purity and beauty, will not occur.

But if parts of the wound have united, and the sutures are holding the flap firmly in place, it does not matter if other parts suppurate, and heal by granulation. Treatment of these areas with silver nitrate will prevent the scar becoming too broad, and in the end it may be as good as if it had healed by first intention. Sometimes, however, scars that are formed in this way tend to contract and leave a depression, whereas scars that result from primary healing give a much smoother transition between the flap and the surrounding skin.

It is not true, as sometimes stated, that wounds in flaps always heal by first intention. But nor is there always infection when transplanted skin is joined to normal skin. It is, however, surprising that primary healing occurs so often in plastic operations, and less often in other operations. The reason for this is that the skin and subcutaneous tissues are ideal for such healing, and other tissues are not often involved.

Dieffenbach notes that healing by granulation is usually rapid in patients who seem to have little capacity for primary healing, whereas wounds with loss of tissue in patients who should heal by first intention are often very slow.[11]

PARTIAL GANGRENE

Sometimes the healing in plastic operations is less certain. A narrow strip at the edge of the flap may slough. As might be expected, this is mostly in the parts furthest from the pedicle—columella, ala, or tip of the nose. It occurs commonly before the whole flap becomes gangrenous, and you need to keep your fingers crossed that the rot does not spread. When a strip has been lost, the defect fills with granulation tissue, and there will be a permanent depressed scar. If the patient is dissatisfied, and there is enough tissue, so that the reconstructed part will not be made too small, the scar can be excised and re-sutured. When the columella has been lost, but the rest of the nose is intact, it can be reconstructed from the upper lip. Sometimes gangrene only affects the outer layers of the flap. It is not easy to tell how deep this has gone, and whether the full thickness of the flap has been destroyed. The only thing to do is to wait patiently until the dead tissue has sloughed off naturally, and not to be in a hurry to remove it. It may then be a pleasant surprise to find that there are good granulations under the scab, so that a deformity will be avoided.

GANGRENE

If there is no healing by the third or fourth day, and the flap is only held in place by the sutures, with pus pouring out, the flap will die. The vessels in the pedicle may not have been adequate to nourish the flap, which remains as pale, cold, and wrinkled as when it was raised. But, more commonly, too much blood has entered the flap, and has not drained naturally through the veins, nor been released artificially. Sometimes the fault lies in the dense scar-tissue in the margins of the defect to which the flap is sutured, or there may be some underlying disease, especially what is simply called 'pyogenesis' (the tendency for the simplest cut to suppurate), and if stimulating treatment is then used, instead of anti-inflammatory treatment, the loss of the flap is hardly surprising. Tagliacozzi noted that gangrene in a flap on the arm is sometimes due to too strong a grip with the forceps by which it is

[11] Dieffenbach, *Erfahrungen,* Vol. 2, p. 71 (1830).

lifted up, or to the bandage being too tight.[12] Both these risks are avoided in the (now much more common) Indian method. Gangrene in a flap is the same process as in any other part, but it is nearly always the dry, and not the moist, type that destroys a flap.

Case history This case history of Dieffenbach's illustrates some of these problems: a healthy 27-year-old journeyman mason was so hideously deformed that people kept out of his way, regarding him as a sinner who carried in his face the marks of his evil deeds. His nose was missing, so that there was just a hole; he had also lost half his upper lip, and the rest of his face was covered with scars. It looked undoubtedly to be the result of syphilis, but the patient swore that he had never been infected, and that a fall from a height at the age of 13 had been followed by gangrene. He seemed an honest fellow, and, at any rate, his robust health showed that there was no residual underlying disease.

Reconstruction was carried out in one stage. The lip was repaired first by a horizontal incision in the remaining half of the upper lip, and wide undermining from the maxilla, so that the lip could be advanced and sutured to the opposite angle of the mouth. Then a flap was taken from the centre of the forehead, with its pedicle between the eyebrows; the columella was made from an inch-wide strip of previously shaved skin at the upper end. The flap was positioned so that its pedicle lay over the region of the bridge of the nose, and the main part covered the rest of the defect. The columella was attached to the upper lip with four interrupted sutures; twelve twisted sutures were used for the nose, and six in the forehead, leaving only a narrow gap in the middle of the forehead. Cold dressings were applied to the forehead, and tepid dressings to the flap. The patient was put on an anti-inflammatory diet, with lemonade and cream of tartar to drink. He was able to sleep a little that night. Apart from a high fever for several days, needing vigorous blood-letting, he was in no danger.

Immediately after the operation the flap was pale, cold, and flaccid, but it gradually became congested, and by the evening it was very swollen and hot, although it was still pale. At 24 hours most of the pins were removed from the flap. On the third day the columella and the tip of the nose were suspiciously blue and cold. Eight leeches were applied to each cheek, but the parts became necrotic at 4–5 days, and could be removed with forceps on the seventh day. In spite of the fact that, at first, union had seemed to be complete, it began to break down at

[12] Tagliacozzi, *de curtorum*, Vol. 2, Chapter 6.

various points. Two-thirds of the wound in the lip separated, but by the ninth day the flap had healed, and the gap in the lip was smaller. The patient was well and cheerful. The wound in the lip was excised and re-sutured, and continuous ice-packs were applied. This left a small hole in the middle of the lip, which was soon healed by touching with cantharides, and pulling together with sticking-plaster. Thus the greater part of his deformity was relieved, but the columella and the tip of his nose were still missing. Dieffenbach proposed to reconstruct these from the left cheek, but the patient proved obstinate, thinking himself lucky enough already. In spite of all persuasion, he denied Dieffenbach the pleasure of improving his appearance still further, and he even refused to have the pedicle of the flap divided. He had been in the Charité from 29 June to 22 August—less than eight weeks.[13]

THE NERVE-SUPPLY OF FLAPS

The influence of the nerves on the success or failure of a flap must now be considered. Sometimes a flap, even with a very narrow pedicle, has only a little less sensation than the rest of the skin. The patient feels the touch of a finger on the flap, or the prick of a needle when it is sutured, almost as distinctly as normal. When a flap has been transplanted from the forehead to the nose, the stimulus is not felt in the nose, but in the forehead, i.e. there is a phantom sensation similar to that after amputation of a limb, where the patient describes so accurately the feeling in the limb, that, even though he can see that it has been amputated, it sounds as if he does not believe it. In the same way, after a major plastic operation, all the stimuli to a flap are felt by the patient at the site from which it was taken. But it also sometimes happens that the sensation is greatly diminished, so that at first the patient feels neither touch nor the prick of a needle. The sensation is always better with a wide pedicle, for then it is more likely that a large nerve will have been included.

The illusory sensation in a flap arises from the fact that we only learn by experience that sensations that are transmitted by the nerves to the sensorium are the result of particular stimuli. If a nerve and the skin which it supplies are now moved to another site, any sensation from it reaching the sensorium is exactly the same as before, and the patient must learn by experience that what feels like a touch on his forehead must have taken place on his new nose. With his eyes closed, he feels a touch on part of the nose, such as the tip, in the exact place on the

[13] Dieffenbach, *Erfahrungen,* Vol. 2, p. 67 (1830).

forehead from which that part came; this disordered sensation gradually disappears. A flap that is at first quite numb will become sensitive again.

Although normal sensation will return to the flap in time, its absence indicates that the influence of the vegetative nervous system is also in abeyance, There is bound to be more anxiety about the nutrition of a freshly transplanted flap if it is insensitive than if it has normal sensation. Lack of nervous influence is one of the factors that sometimes contributes to the loss of a flap. In this context, Gräfe noticed after a forehead rhinoplasty that, during the time that sensation in the flap was completely absent, the processes of granulation and scarring were extremely active.[14]

PHOTOPHOBIA AFTER A FLAP FROM THE FOREHEAD

In reading the plastic surgical literature I have never come across a description of this physiologically interesting phenomenon.[15] In several nasal reconstructions by von Ammon, and in one of my own, the patients complained of the intolerable glare of the light, immediately after the separation of the flap from the forehead, at a time when the sunlight was not particularly strong; in my case, the day was so gloomy that there was hardly enough light for the operation. There was no relief when the patient closed his eyes, nor when I covered the wound on the forehead with a sponge. I had to allow the patient to turn away from the light from time to time; this prolonged an already difficult operation. The troublesome symptom disappeared spontaneously as soon as the patient was back in bed, and it did not recur. I do not know the explanation for this, nor how to protect the patient from it; turning him away from the window is not always practicable, as it takes away the light needed to finish the operation.

A wound so near the eyes must increase their sensitivity, but operations which are even nearer, such as blepharoplasty, do not produce photophobia. Also, it does not happen in every forehead rhinoplasty, and it resolves quickly. It seems most likely that it is caused by injury to nerves close to the eye, either at the glabella or the root of the nose.

---

[14] C. F. von Gräfe, Fall von Rhinoplastik aus der Stirn, *J. Chir. Augenheilk.* **12,** 11 (1828).

[15] [Zeis was the first to describe this.]

ERYSIPELAS

Erysipelas is very common after plastic operations, particularly on the face. The trauma of the operation, the undermining of large pieces of skin, and the number of sutures predispose to it in the first few days after operation. Sometimes it is only an erysipelas-like inflammation, but more often it is the true erysipelas. If the patient has had previous attacks, even on the foot, or has a tendency to it, especially with a delicate, irritable skin, and if careful preliminary treatment to clean the intestine has not been carried out, then any plastic operation on the face is likely to be followed by erysipelas. This is sometimes bullous, and it may spread over the scalp and the greater part of the back. Sometimes it spreads out from the flap, and sometimes from the surrounding skin into the flap.

The onset of erysipelas prevents the use of wet dressings, and interferes with primary healing. A strong emetic is the only way of checking it, but, after a rhinoplasty, this may be contraindicated by the risk that violent retching may tear the delicate new adhesions of the flap. Gentle cooling treatment must then be used, with care to prevent the fever reaching a dangerous level.

There are times, particularly in scarlet fever epidemics, when erysipelas seems to be contagious. I once saw eight or ten patients with various eye diseases and surgical conditions, after operation, or waiting for operation, all attacked together. When contagious erysipelas rages in a hospital, every blood-letting, leech-bite, wound, and scratch is affected. With the greatest cleanliness, and avoidance of the foul habit of washing all ulcers and wounds with the same sponge, the disease can be controlled, except on those wards which do not observe these precautions.

In one of Gräfe's cases of rhinoplasty, erysipelas started in the new nose on the fourth day, and spread out over the face and scalp with severe headache and swinging fever. The nose became livid, hot, and blistered. Gräfe advised against local treatment with stimulants, antiseptics, and warming, which are always to be avoided when the flap is hot, because they cause accumulation of fluid and slowing of the circulation. Instead he recommended blood-letting, acid aperients, cream of tartar to drink, and local compresses of lead lotion; soon the dangerous symptoms abated.[16]

Dieffenbach described similar cases, so that it is ludicrous for Blandin to stress the fact that the nose in one of his patients was attacked by

[16] C. F. von Gräfe, Fall von Rhinoplastik, *J. Chir. Augenheilk.* **13,** 2 (1829).

erysipelas six weeks after the operation, whereas a nose made by Dieffenbach did not go yellow when the patient became jaundiced six months after operation.[17] Blandin attributes this striking difference to the excellence of his technique, by which he ensures that there are as many blood-vessels as possible in the flap, so that his noses are better nourished and healthier. But he does not realize that German noses, unfortunately, are also attacked early and often by erysipelas, and that his comparison of erysipelas and jaundice is pointless because they are different diseases.

MUCOUS MEMBRANE

Mucous membrane is much less well adapted for transplantation than skin. Not only is it thinner, so that it cannot be shaped, but its biological properties make it less satisfactory for plastic operations. Even a minor injury causes such a strong reaction that the resulting inflammation is more catarrhal than adhesive, with an increased secretion of mucus; this inflammation is greater than is needed for primary healing. Tagliacozzi knew that it was more difficult to get a flap from the arm to unite to the mucous membrane of the nose than to the skin.[18] However, it is sometimes necessary to transplant pieces of mucous membrane, either to make the part as natural as possible, such as the lip and the eyelid which must be lined with mucous membrane, or to reconstruct a part which, because of its site, cannot be replaced by skin, such as the palate, i.e. staphyloplasty rather than staphylorrhaphy.[19] The smaller the piece the easier it is to transplant. Plastic surgery has been greatly advanced by Dieffenbach's technique of lining the margins of an opening, such as the mouth, with mucous membrane, to prevent recurrence of a contracture.[20]

Sometimes a flap is transplanted in such a way that the outer surface becomes the inner, and the mucosal surface is on the outside, as in reconstruction of the columella from the upper lip, where a flap is taken from the full thickness of the lip, and turned directly upwards. It is interesting to see how the mucous membrane is changed by prolonged contact with the air—it stops secreting, and becomes as dry as skin; the epithelium changes to epidermis, and its dark-red colour becomes paler and more like skin. On closer examination there are still perma-

[17] Blandin, *Autoplastie,* p. 202.

[18] Tagliacozzi, *de curtorum,* Vol. 2, Chapter 15.

[19] [See p. 171, n. 1.]

[20] [See p. 163, n. 6.]

nent differences—the mucous membrane looks more like a scar, it is smoother, without the little folds in normal skin, and there are no hairs or sebaceous glands. The same changes are seen in mucous membrane which becomes dry from lack of saliva when exposed to the air by disease, as in the gums when the lips or cheeks are destroyed.

Conversely, skin changes to become more like mucous membrane when it is kept away from the air, but in contact with another skin surface. This happens in every skin fold, as with the chafing of the deep folds in small fat children. Dieffenbach also reported it in a successful case of reconstruction of the foreskin from the skin of the penis. The skin that had been turned in towards the glans became red and moist with secretion. Although it was known that mucous membrane, and even serous membranes, take on the appearance of skin when exposed to the air, no one before him had observed that skin, out of contact with the air, changes into a secreting membrane. The secretion was not sweat, and it did not come from the glans, which was almost dry.[21]

ANATOMICAL STUDIES

There are very few dissections of reconstructed parts. I once carried out a post-mortem on a woman who had had her nose and one eyelid reconstructed. There were no major changes in the transplanted skin, and the scar tissue was the same as in other scars. With the loupe the skin was seen to contain more whiteish tendinous fibres than normal reddish-yellow skin. There was no opportunity to inject the head to demonstrate the vessels supplying the flap.

The only observation of this kind is by von Walther—a 34-year-old man lost his nose from syphilis, and it had been reconstructed from the forehead. The nose was flat because it had no support, and the patient stuffed it with blotting-paper. Some time later this wretch was executed for murder. Dissection of the injected head showed the following: the skin over the nasal bones was covered with black hair. The dermis and superficial fascia were markedly thickened, and attached to the latter were the fibres of the muscle excised from the forehead. The new nose was richly supplied with arteries—branches of the external maxillary (facial) and ophthalmic arteries, with branches from the coronary artery of the upper lip and the angular artery giving many twigs to the ala, and spreading out laterally and towards the bridge of the nose.[22]

[21] [See p. 184.]

[22] Von Walther, Wiederanheilung, p. 530 (1825).

9

THE CARE OF THE PATIENT AFTER OPERATION

GRÄFE'S REGIME

Gräfe has given very detailed instructions for the care of the patient.[1] In a favourable case after operation, bodily functions are normal, there is adhesive inflammation, and the edges of the wound are moderately congested and covered with yellowish fibrin. The surgeon then has little to do, except to ensure that the patient does not become constipated, leading to congestion of the head. If the inflammation is more severe, becoming synochal,[2] all anti-inflammatory measures must be undertaken, even blood-letting, with nitrum,[3] gentle aperients and cool drinks, and the room kept cool. If inflammation reaches the erethistic stage,[4] there is severe pain in the face and arm (in the German method), the patient cannot sleep, and he has a small, rapid pulse and an anxious look; the wound is swollen, but not as tense as in the previous stage. Gangrene is then to be feared. Treatment is by opium with saltpetre, extract of henbane,[5] cherry-laurel water[6] with almond-milk, and sometimes blood-letting; compresses of cold *lotio plumbi* and dressings of lead- or zinc ointment are used instead of local stimulants. Gräfe also gives instructions for the indolent wound, but it appears that he has never seen this in transplanted tissue, and his description is taken from observations on other wounds. At the very beginning, Gräfe's regime is stimulating: *Balsam Commendatoris*,[7] aromatic wool, and spirit lotions, on the assumption that a flap needs such treatment to keep it alive. Only when true inflammation sets in does he advise an antiphlogistic regime (including blood-letting), but not the vigorous use of cold on the

[1] Gräfe, *Rhinoplastik*, pp. 55, 95, 146, 160.
[2] [With continued fever.]
[3] [Saltpetre (potassium nitrate), a febrifuge.]
[4] [Febris nervosa, increased sensitivity of the nervous system.]
[5] [*Hyoscyamus niger*.]
[6] [*Prunus laurocerasus*.]
[7] [Tinct. benz. co.]

flap. This (like his operation) is all much more complicated than the regime that Dieffenbach recommends, and which many other surgeons now follow with excellent results.

DIEFFENBACH'S REGIME

Dieffenbach's management is based on a very different view of the physiology of a wound. Like the more recent treatment of gangrene, which does not use antiseptics on the dead tissue, but directs all attention to stopping the progress of the gangrene in the still-living, but inflamed, tissues, Dieffenbach treats the part to which the flap is attached. In addition, he uses the Indian method much more often than the Italian, and attaches the flap with his twisted sutures,[8] so that there is no need for the complicated dressings of Tagliacozzi's and Gräfe's methods. Apart from a dressing on the forehead, no other is used; even the sticking-plaster between the sutures is not needed, as the twisted sutures hold the flap firmly. This has the advantage of allowing uninterrupted observation of the progress of the flap. There is no raw surface to be protected from the air, for the flap is covered with epidermis, and the twisted threads cover the wound edges. Recent experience, and better observation of the reunion of completely separated parts, have shown, as Montégre first reported,[9] that a delay before reattachment is advantageous. This proves that the danger of the death of a flap (which is in any case not completely separated) is nowhere near as great as was first thought at the revival of *chirurgia curtorum* in the present century.

GENERAL MANAGEMENT

Patients who have had plastic operations do not usually suffer from loss of blood, but from exhaustion due to pain. The length of the operation, particularly when twisted sutures are used, means that, by the end, they are pale and cold, and it is time to get them back to bed. The flap shows the effects of this reduced peripheral circulation: it is pale and limp, and it does not project like a nose, but covers the nasal cavity like a piece of cloth. But after an hour or so, when the patient has had some sleep, and drunk several cups of tea, the normal temperature returns, and then all too easily rises higher than is desirable. In the certainty that this will happen, cold compresses are applied liberally to the flap

[8] [See p. 102, n. 38.]

[9] [See p. 18, n. 1.]

and its donor area immediately after the end of the operation. Although the healing of the donor area by suppuration and granulation cannot be avoided, inflammation here must be controlled, in case it spreads to the flap. The cold dressings relieve the pain in the forehead, which is due to the tension of pulling the skin together to reduce the size of the defect, and which, before the inflammatory reaction sets in, is the only thing that the patient feels.

On the day of the operation, the patient should be in good general health, and have had his bowels open. All that is then needed after the operation is to give warming drinks for some hours to raise the skin temperature, and to administer neutral salts or a weak acid, with lemonade or cream of tartar to drink. The patient soon finds that this regime is doing him good, and requests the frequent renewal of the cold compresses; in spite of these, it is common to find the flap red and slightly swollen by the evening. In the first few days after operation, little change in this regime is needed. After a rhinoplasty the tubes in the nostrils, which allow the passage of air, must be kept clean, and after blepharoplasty the exudate must be removed from the eye. The dressing on the donor area should be left undisturbed for several days, until it has been lifted by pus, so that its removal is easy. For the next dressing, the lint is smeared with a mild ointment to prevent it sticking. If the granulations are too high, the raw surface is touched with silver nitrate to encourage it to contract. As the sutures are gradually removed, sticking-plaster is applied, as necessary, but this provides only slight support for the suture-line. If the flap has been taken from a part of the body that is normally kept covered, it must be allowed to get brown in the sun, so that it will match its surroundings; this is unnecessary after the Indian operation. Hair on the flap should be plucked until it stops growing.

If the case is proceeding normally, the surgeon can play a fairly passive role, keeping a careful watch for complications. Local blood-letting and the vigorous use of cold on a blue swollen flap have already been discussed.[10] It is possible that a flap may sometimes need mild local stimulation with warm aromatic fomentations, aromatic cotton wool, and spirituous applications. This is not to be condemned outright, but it should not be used routinely; I have never seen a case that needed it. There is no doubt that Dieffenbach's more natural method of after-care has given excellent results, which have contributed to the dissemination of plastic surgery.

---

[10] See p. 70.

High fever and other major complications require the most diligent care, but they are managed on general surgical principles, which will not be discussed here, as I assume that they are well known.

10

GENERAL OPERATIVE TECHNIQUE

RECONSTRUCTION BY COMPLETELY SEPARATED PIECES OF SKIN

Missing parts can be reconstructed by completely or incompletely separated pieces of skin. But the healing of a completely separated piece of skin, either on the same bed, or on some other site, even if sometimes successful, is so unreliable that it cannot be recommended for routine practice. Further attempts should certainly be made so that the subject can be studied. This is a method of rhinoplasty that is said to be practised in India, but it has not been taken up in Europe. Apart from Bünger's case,[1] and Dieffenbach's experiments with pieces of skin on the arm[2] (which were not done for any therapeutic purpose), there are only Dzondi's cases, which were also unsuccessful. He reconstructed part of a woman's left nostril, which had been destroyed by infection.

The skin was taken from the lower hairless border of the left hand of a young student, who willingly volunteered. The site was beaten with a rod of whale-bone for half an hour beforehand to make it inflamed. While this was being done, the margins of the defect were prepared. Dzondi then measured the defect, and cut a piece of skin to this size from the hand, in the shape of a rhomboid, a quarter of an inch wide in the centre. He folded it into a triangle with the raw surfaces together, and fixed it into the defect with sticking plaster. For the first three days there was no sign of pus, but then suppuration set in. When the discoloured piece of skin had to be removed, Dzondi found that a thin strip had united to the upper edge of the nostril, so that its removal caused pain and bleeding. This operation had a happy outcome for the patient, for the defect became filled with granulation tissue, and she was completely restored.[3] This was clearly too big a procedure for a defect that was small enough to be obliterated simply by granulation tissue.

---

[1] See p. 21, n. 20.

[2] See p. 25, n. 30.

[3] C. H. Dzondi, Ersatz des linken Nasenflügels, *Magazin ges. Heilk.* **6**, 1 (1819).

Another attempted transplantation by Dzondi, from the upper arm to the calf, and vice versa, failed; he thought that this was because the areas had not been brought to an inflammatory state beforehand. In a second unsuccessful case, in a patient weakened by syphilis, the site on the upper arm, which had been beaten with whalebone, gave much less pain than the site on the thigh, which had only been rubbed by hand.[4]

Thus the two possibilities for transplanting completely separated pieces of skin are to take them either from the same individual (Bünger's operation), or from someone else (Dzondi).

TRANSPLANTING INCOMPLETELY SEPARATED PIECES OF SKIN

A flap of incompletely separated skin remains attached to its site of origin, from which it is not divided until it has united with its new site. It, too, can be taken from the same or from another individual. The latter procedure is conceivable, and could perhaps be carried out. But 6–8 days are needed before a flap can be safely divided, and there would be very great difficulties in keeping two people in such close contact for this length of time without damage to the flap.

There are two ways of taking a flap from the same individual: from a distance (the Italian method) or from nearby (the more common Indian method). In the former, the flap is either raised and allowed to contract before it is transplanted, or it is attached as soon as it has been raised.

ATTACHING THE FLAP BY ITS MARGINS OR BY ITS UNDER-SURFACE

There are sites, both in the Italian and the Indian methods, where the flap can only be attached by its margins, e.g. rhinoplasty, cheiloplasty, and otoplasty. It is then only nourished by the vessels which penetrate the scar at the margins (in the Indian method, by the pedicle as well). In a rhinoplasty the flap is stretched over a cavity, to which its inner surface can find no attachment. This raw surface therefore becomes scarred, which is just what is wanted, for the scar contracts and pushes the flap forward, giving it prominence, and there is no tendency for it to become adherent. This lack of adhesion would be highly desirable in other cases, such as cheiloplasty, where the flap may adhere to the gum, so that movements of the jaw are restricted. It is very hard to prevent these adhesions forming, or to prevent their recurrence when they are divided.

---

[4] Ibid. p. 11.

But there are also many plastic operations where the aim is to get the under-surface of the flap to adhere, but where it is as difficult to achieve this as, in other cases, to prevent it. The closure of urinary fistulae is often delayed by the failure of the skin of the penis (more than any other type of skin) to adhere to its new bed. In the repair of some parts of the nose it is often the intention that the flap should heal to the underlying tissues. But healing by the margins is quicker; the adhesion of the under-surface comes later, and must be promoted by gentle stimulating injections into the cavity or pocket under the flap.

PREPARATION OF A PEDICLED FLAP

A flap is a piece of skin, usually square, which has been freed on three sides, and from its bed, leaving one side intact through which it is nourished. This attachment (the pedicle) may be as broad as the flap itself, as in the Italian method, or much narrower, to allow the flap to rotate, as in the Indian method. In the Italian method, rotation is not necessary, as the flap is designed on the arm so that it goes straight on to the face; for a nose, the flap retains its attachment to the arm near the elbow, and, for a lower lip, near the shoulder. In the Indian method, rotation cannot usually be avoided, although there are various ways of bringing the flap closer to the defect. In making a nose, the flap remains attached near the root of the nose between the eyebrows. If it is not free enough, parallel incisions, one inch apart, are carried a little way down on to the bridge of the nose, until, by repeated testing, there is no tension when the flap is rotated. This pedicle is much narrower than in the Italian method, and care must be taken that the degree of rotation does not obstruct the circulation of blood. A width of one inch is usually enough; when the forehead is scarred it should be broader.

INSETTING THE PEDICLE

The descriptions of the operation by the Indian surgeons do not give enough details to show how they dealt with the pedicle. Carpue and Gräfe laid it over the skin on the bridge of the nose. Naturally, there is no adhesion between its raw surface and the intact skin. They, and their followers, then excised the pedicle when the flap was completely healed, to make the surface level. A sound was passed under it, and it was divided. The lower border was sutured to the edge of the defect on the bridge of the nose. They tried to return the upper part to the forehead or the glabella, but, because the healing in this area was already advanced, or even complete, this was not usually practicable.

One of Dieffenbach's greatest services to plastic surgery is his modification of this procedure, which makes the Indian method even easier and more certain of success. He was the first to extend one of the incisions for the pedicle down over the bridge of the nose as far as the defect.[5] The edges of this incision retract, or they can be undermined, so that there is enough room for the pedicle to lie in the gap. This makes the rotation of the flap easier, so that the pedicle can be broader than with the earlier method. There is also the advantage that the pedicle unites with the skin edges and with its bed, giving the flap a much greater blood-supply. Excision of the prominence caused by the rotation of the pedicle is still necessary, but the lump is not as big as before. There is no need to lift the pedicle from its bed or to divide it completely—only a small ellipse of skin, the shape of a myrtle leaf, is excised, and often most of it can be left permanently. This principle of rotating and insetting the pedicle is, of course, applicable, not only to rhinoplasty, but to all other local flaps.

Labat and Blandin, in common with other French surgeons, regard all secondary operations in plastic surgery as unnecessary and unjustifiable, and they would ban these procedures in patients who have lost their nerve after the agonies of the first operation. By stopping half-way like this, they leave their patients without even having the pedicle excised, and they do not regard the residual lump as a deformity.[6] Blandin is clearly against its excision,[7] allowing it only for the cases where the flap has to be brought from a distance. At the same time he criticizes Dieffenbach's procedure for insetting the pedicle. Like all his countrymen, he pays no attention to anything that comes from abroad, and regards everything new and good as a French discovery. But then he contradicts himself by recommending (as a discovery by Lisfranc for rhinoplasty, and by Lallemand for cheiloplasty) that one of the incisions for the pedicle should be extended down to the defect.[8] This is exactly the same as Dieffenbach's technique, which he has condemned. But, more than that, he recommends a technique of his

---

[5] Dieffenbach, *Erfahrungen*, Vol. 2, p. 32 (1830).

[6] But as Tagliacozzi reminds us: 'there is nothing that is perfect at first. Rome was not built in a day. All human achievements must be attained by slow steps up to the summit of perfection. In this way all arts and knowledge have grown.' *de curtorum*, Vol. 2, Chapter 7, p. 21.

[7] La section du pédicule du lambeau qui a servi à l'autoplastie doit être abandonnée, *Autoplastie*, p. 124.

[8] '. . . par le prolongement de l'une de ces incisions destinées à circonscrire le lambeau jusqu'à cette solution, l'autre en demeurant éloignée de toute l'épaisseur du pédicule.' ibid, p. 127.

own: that the skin of the nasal bridge should be incised later, and the pedicle then inset.[9] Not only is it much more difficult to make an incision when the pedicle is lying on the nose, but its margins and under-surface have become scarred, and are thus less likely to unite with the bed. This simply gives the same result as Dieffenbach's method, but more slowly and less safely.

ROTATION OF THE FLAP

In the Indian method, as practised by Carpue and Gräfe, it is immaterial whether the flap is rotated to the right or the left. But with Dieffenbach's technique of insetting the pedicle, the direction of rotation must be decided before the incision is extended down the nose. If the rotation is to be to the patient's right, the incision on the right of the pedicle is extended [Fig. 6], and vice versa. For the surgeon it is usually easier if the flap is rotated to the left, i.e. to his right.

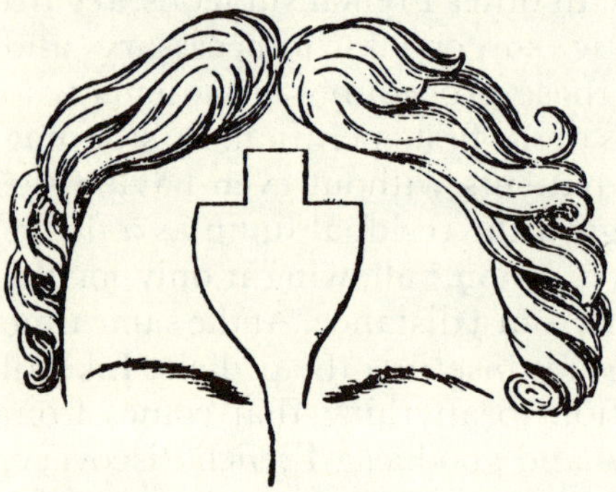

Fig. 6

If the flap is taken vertically from the middle of the forehead it must be rotated through 180°. This is the maximum rotation, and in many cases it can be less. When the forehead is scarred, the flap can be taken obliquely from one side; the incision is then extended accordingly, and the rotation is about 140° [Fig. 7]. In other cases, e.g. von Ammon's cheiloplasty,[10] the rotation is only 90°.

The rule, then, is that the incision is carried down to the defect on the side to which the flap is to be rotated [Fig. 8]: if a flap, *a*, is to be laid into a defect, *b*, it is the incision *d*, and not *c*, that must be continued to the point *e*, so that the flap can rotate along the dotted line *f*. It is very important that the rotation is kept as small as possible, to reduce compression of the vessels in the pedicle, and to improve the flow of blood into and, more particularly, out of the flap.

But there are other factors which can make the rotation less than 180°: with a low forehead, it is often not possible to make the columella, or even the tip of the nose, except by using hairy scalp; this can be

[9] Ibid. pp. 172ff.
[10] See p. 160.

partly overcome by laying the pattern obliquely on the forehead (although repeated plucking can make even hairy skin suitable for rhinoplasty). Again, if one flap from the forehead has failed, and the Italian method is not to be used, a second flap may be taken obliquely. If there is scarring on one side, which encroaches on the site of the flap, the inevitable contracture may distort the eyebrow or even the eyelid. Injury to the supraorbital nerve is also cited as a contraindication to the oblique operation. It has been said that its division may be very dangerous, with inevitable blindness; but injuries to it are common without such complications. The question whether division really causes blindness has not yet been decided, In two cases of von Ammon's the flap was taken from the side of the forehead, and injury to the nerve was unavoidable, but there was not the slightest effect on vision. It is the same with reconstruction of the upper eyelid—it has never been known to be followed by blindness. The danger has been exaggerated, and it is not a contraindication to taking the flap from the side of the forehead.

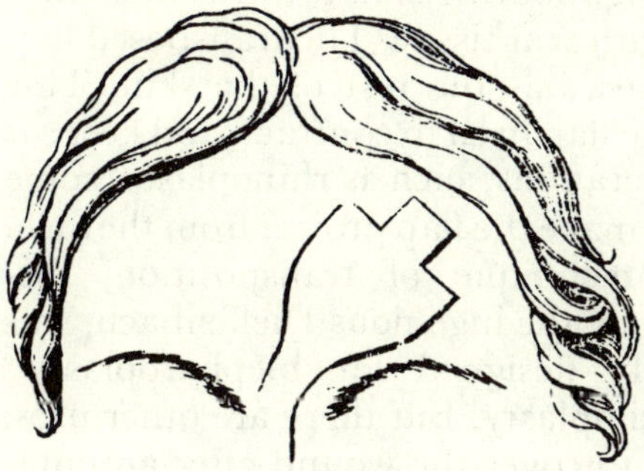

Fig. 7

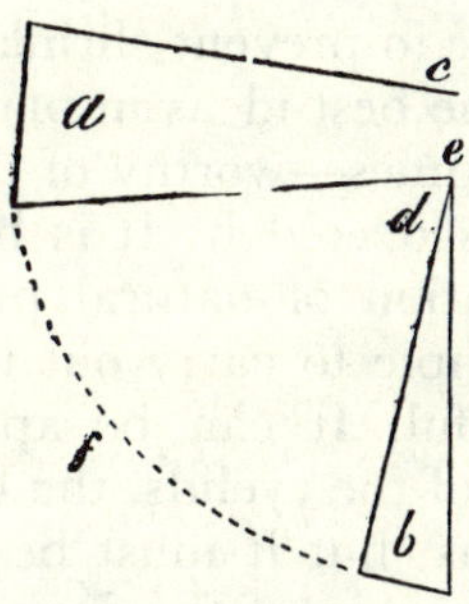

Fig. 8

TRANSPOSITION OF THE FLAP

The more acute the angle through which the flap is turned the nearer the technique comes to transposition.[11]

To fill the defect *a* the flap *b* is taken from adjoining skin. One side of the defect *c* is already one edge of the flap, which does not have to be lifted over intact skin [Fig. 9]. The pedicle needs only 30–40° rotation, and can therefore be broader than when the rotation is greater. Such a small rotation causes no heaping up of the skin, so that a secondary operation is unnecessary.

[11] [lit. 'sideways shifting of the flap'.]

The flap *b* is now in the defect, with the raw area, *a*, immediately next to it [Fig. 10]. The edges of the flap, *c* and *f*, are sutured in place. The corner of the flap, *d*, is now where the angle *e* of the defect was.

The characteristic of this operation is that it leaves a contracting scar immediately adjacent to the flap. Contracture of a scar is Nature's way of healing a defect by pulling the neighbouring skin towards it, so that the whole area is not simply filled with scar tissue. The transposed flap is put under tension in the same way as the rest of the skin. This counteracts the great tendency of the flap itself to contract, and keeps it stretched out smoothly. In other operations, such as rhinoplasty, some degree of contracture is desirable to make the flap project from the face.

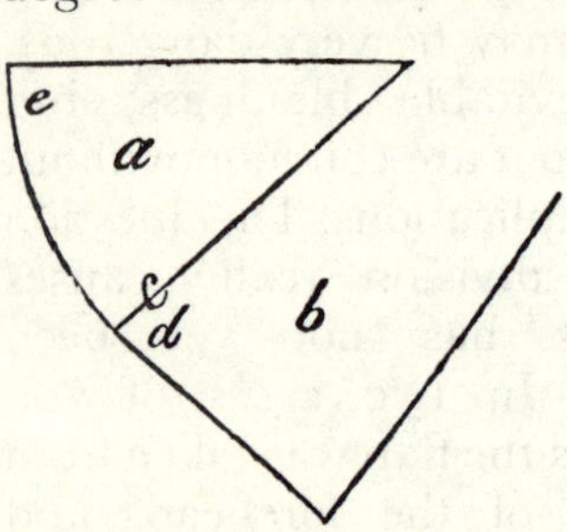

Fig. 9

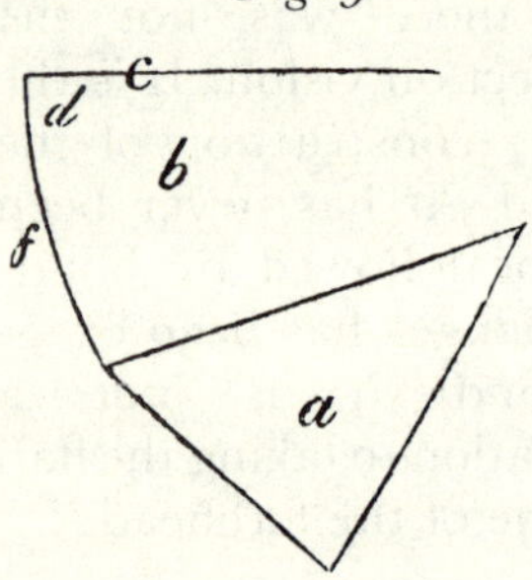

Fig. 10

The technique of transposition, discovered by the ingenious Dieffenbach, was originally designed for blepharoplasty[12] and cheiloplasty. But there are other uses, such as to cover the wound after amputation of the breast, as a possible way of preventing recurrence.[13] The use of a contracting scar to prevent shrinkage of a flap is one of the best ideas in plastic surgery in recent times—worthy of the great master who discovered it. It is based on careful observation of natural processes, and it is so simple to carry out that it is always successful. It can be applied to reconstruction of the eyelids, the lips, and other operations, but it must be obvious that, even if the skin of the face near the nose were suitable for a rhinoplasty, this method could not be used to replace the whole nose, as it is only designed to repair flat defects.

ADVANCEMENT OF SKIN

Another method that is useful in many cases is advancement [Fig. 11]. If the rectangle *a* is a defect, and at *b* there is an excess of skin, this can be raised as a flap, advanced as far as possible, and sutured *cc* to *dd* and at the sides. This technique was often used to close fistulae, particularly

---

[12] [See p. 137, n. 11.]

[13] [See p. 178, n, 1.]

of the urethra. Failure was not due to the method, but to the fact that it needs more to close a fistula. When only the outer layer of skin has been repaired, the internal opening still remains; permeation of urine continues (even when a catheter is used), and this prevents the flap from uniting. The principle of advancement can also be used when the edge of the flap *cc* cannot be sutured to *dd*, and the flap is only retained in its new site by the lateral sutures. This was one method of cheiloplasty, where the edge *cc* formed the free border of the lip, but this flap retracted so much that the results were very poor. It is more suitable for flat surfaces, especially after excision of scars, when there is not enough skin simply to be pulled together.

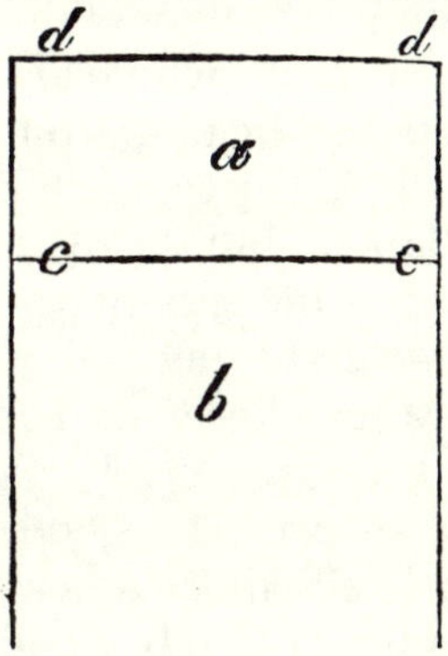

Fig. 11

BUILDING UP SUNKEN PARTS

All attempts to improve the shape of a reconstructed part by any sort of external splinting are useless. When the apparatus is removed, the skin keeps its new shape for a while, but then follows the natural laws of contraction. Dieffenbach was the first to introduce an operative technique—this is mainly used for the nose.[14]

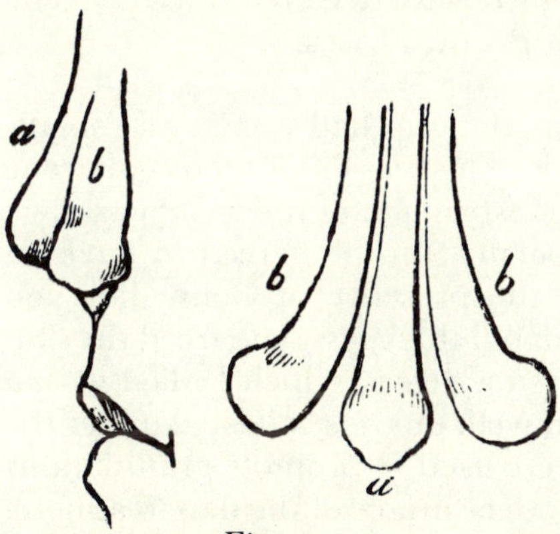

Fig. 12

If the bony and cartilaginous supports of the nose have been destroyed (but the skin is intact), the skin is divided into flaps, where *a* represents the bridge and *b b* the side-walls of the nose [Fig. 12]. The edges of these flaps are cut obliquely, so that more tissue is removed from the posterior surface, and none from the epidermal surface. The flaps then become like vault-stones, wider on one side and narrower on the other; when they are sutured together they create a convexity, and lift the sunken nose. If a concavity is needed, as where the side-wall of the nose reaches the face, the flaps should be narrower on the epidermal side and wider at the back. Although no new tissue has

[14] Dieffenbach, *Erfahrungen*, Vol. 1, p. 9 (1829).

been transplanted, this operation may quite correctly be regarded as plastic surgery.

The nose will collapse again if it is not supported. The best way to do this is to run long thick needles through the cheeks under the floor of the nose. Small discs of lead or hard leather are put on the ends, which are twisted up until the nose reaches the desired projection. The pain from the needles is not too bad, but the pressure of the discs is tiresome for the patient. The nose becomes very swollen and inflamed, but the discs withstand the pressure. The needles are left in as long as the patient can tolerate them—for several days or even a week—in the hope that inflammation in the needle tracks will produce strands of scar tissue, which will contract and hold the nose forwards.

Immediately after the operation the results are surprisingly good, but this procedure seems to be less valuable than Dieffenbach's next three techniques. The tendency of the skin to contract, and to become adherent to the underlying tissues, spoils the effect once healing has taken place and the supports have been removed.

INSETTING THE FLAP[15]

Dieffenbach described this technique for the reconstruction of part of an organ, such as the bridge of the nose or one ala, using a pedicled flap and twisted sutures like other plastic operations. There are no rules for the design of the flap, and each case must be treated on its merits.[16] The principle can be illustrated by one of my own cases:

Case report In 1831 a young journeyman tailor had very severe smallpox (although he had been inoculated). This was followed by gangrene of the face and caries of the maxilla; destruction of the nasal cartilage left him with a saddle-nose. With persuasion, he agreed to have an operation. On 22 August 1836, in the presence of Councillor von Ammon, I split the nose lengthways in full thickness, and freed the skin from its deep attachments; this created a defect, which I filled with a small forehead flap. The edges healed well, but pus collected under the flap; irrigations with silver nitrate were used to promote granulations in the cavity, and to encourage the under-surface of the flap to adhere. The defect in the forehead was small enough to be sutured, but the wound suppurated, and healed by granulation after several weeks. Five

[15] ['*Einpflanzung*'—the term used by Dieffenbach for partial reconstruction, as opposed to '*Anpflanzung*', the construction of a completely new part.]

[16] Dieffenbach, *Erfahrungen*, Vol. 3, p. 32 (1834).

weeks after the first operation, I excised the pedicle, and 10 days later I reduced the flap, which I had deliberately made too big. Both wounds suppurated, and the latter took 3–4 weeks to heal.

He was left with a level bridge to his nose, but the flap was still a little prominent, because the skin of the forehead was thicker than the skin of the nose. The forehead was not only thick, but full of sebaceous follicles, which I have always found to be the best sort of skin for transplantation. I decided not to reduce the flap any further, but to wait for the natural disappearance of the swelling—which Carpue wrongly calls oedema.[17] This is indeed what happened, and it would have ruined the result if I had excised any more tissue from the flap. The patient, who had been so hideously deformed through no fault of his own, was delighted with the result. He has now been seen by Professor Dieffenbach and many other surgeons.

LAYING-ON THE FLAP[18]

In all plastic operations it is the rule that as much tissue as possible should be retained. The human body is sacred, and nothing more should be removed from it than is absolutely necessary. It would be criminal to amputate a limb at a higher level than safety requires. In the same way, a patient with a disfigurement of his nose, where the supporting skeleton is undamaged, will be ill served if the nose is amputated, and a complete rhinoplasty is carried out. If the flap were to die, the patient would be much worse off than before. By covering the skeleton with new skin, the nose will be far better than with a full reconstruction, where the cartilage can never be restored. One of Dieffenbach's cases illustrates this technique:

Case report A young man had his face so scarred by scrofula that he looked as if he had been attacked by a flock of crows. Only the lowest part of his nose was unaffected. Dieffenbach decided to cover the whole nose with skin, as one would re-cover a chair. The forehead flap was very thick; it never lost its colour, and, when it had been completely raised, it became as red as a turkey's wattles. On the third day it was very tense, and leeches were applied. By the seventh day, apart from stitch-abscesses on one side, union was proceeding satisfactorily, but the patient developed a severe gastric fever. Dieffenbach would not risk

[17] See p. 49.

[18] ['*Aufpflanzung*'—Dieffenbach's term for covering a deformed nose with skin when the skeleton is intact.]

damage to the flap by giving emetics. There were signs of nervous involvement, with mastoiditis and discharge of pus from the ear, and the patient died. At post-mortem there was a collection of pus between the meninges.[19]

BURYING THE FLAP[20]

Another of Dieffenbach's discoveries is the use of a forehead flap to improve the shape of the collapsed upper part of the bridge of the nose. This operation starts as an 'insetting',[21] but the flap does not remain on the surface. When it is soundly healed, its outer layer is removed by small repeated excisions, and the edges of the wound are closed over the thickened and hardened deeper layers. Thus the flap forms a support, representing bone and cartilage.[22] Dieffenbach splits the dorsum of the nose in its full length to the tip, and frees the skin on both sides from the bone. He fills the defect with a forehead flap, which contracts to form a raised bridge to the nose, with the pedicle sticking out like a horn at its upper border. This projection is freed and inset to raise the upper part of the bridge. Later, he excises narrow strips from the flap in stages; this brings the bridge level. Every flap forms a thick solid mass, so that here, after removal of its outer layer, the tissue that is left is almost cartilaginous. The skin of the nose is brought together over this and sutured. From the outside, the flap is invisible, but its buried part carries out the function of the nasal bones.

FOLDING THE FLAP

A flap can only be buried if it has already completely healed into place, especially on its under-surface. If a freshly raised flap is placed in a pocket under another piece of skin it will always suppurate. If skin is brought together over a flap its raw surface will not adhere to the epidermis of the flap; the epidermis must first be removed, and this will destroy the flap unless it has already united to its bed. These are the reasons for doubting the practicality of the operation that Blandin[23] attributes to Velpeau: folding a square flap lengthways on itself, or from side to side, and using this to fill a fistula, held in place with a few

[19] Dieffenbach, *Erfahrungen*, Vol. 3, p. 46 (1834).

[20] ['*Unterpflanzung*'—Dieffenbach's term for burying a flap to act as a support.]

[21] See n. 15 above.

[22] Dieffenbach, *Erfahrungen*, Vol. 2, p. 104 (1830); Vol. 3, p. 52 (1834).

[23] Blandin, *Autoplastie*, p. 154.

sutures.[24] This is technically easy, but the difficulty must be to get it to heal. I have no personal experience of this, but it seems inevitable that such a flap would be destroyed by suppuration in a fresh wound, let alone in a chronic fistula.

Jameson, in Baltimore, is said to have used a similar technique for the successful cure of hernias,[25] and Blandin thinks that it could be used to close an artificial anus. But this is not new, for Dzondi has already implanted a skin flap in the inguinal ring.[26]

UNROLLING A FLAP

The unrolling of a flap which has become rolled up is not actually a plastic operation. But in a vesico-vaginal fistula it is usual to replace the torn flap of vagina before attempting any other form of closure. In many of his cases, Dieffenbach was pleased to find a flap of vaginal mucosa curled up near the fistula. Less careful observers might have thought that there was a deficiency of tissue, and used another piece of the mucous membrane to replace it. But in Dieffenbach's cases, even after a long time (in one case, 17 years), the torn strip could be unrolled and sutured back into place.

LINING AN OPENING WITH MUCOUS MEMBRANE TO PREVENT CONTRACTURE

To prevent recurrent contracture of a scarred mouth that has been opened up, Dieffenbach advised that more mucous membrane should be preserved than skin, so that the skin could be hemmed round its edge, like a shoe, with the mucous membrane. The difficulties of transplanting mucous membrane have already been described,[27] but when smaller pieces are simply advanced, and not raised as flaps, this almost always succeeds. Here, interrupted sutures are better than twisted sutures, where the points of the pins excoriate the opposite lip.

DOUBLING THE EDGES OF A FLAP TO PREVENT THEM CONTRACTING

One of the great problems in all plastic operations is contracture of the flap. This can be countered by making the flap bigger than necessary. But this does not prevent the edges contracting when they are left free,

---

[24] See p. 176.
[25] See p. 199, n. 4.
[26] See p. 199, n. 2.
[27] See p. 78.

without being sutured. This is much more marked than in other parts of the flap, particularly at the margins of the nostrils and the free borders of the eyelid and the lip. Dieffenbach's new methods for reconstructing the eyelid and the lip have done away with the need for the procedure described below. In any case, it cannot be applied to the eyelid, for the globe would be in danger of severe irritation if the epidermal surface of the skin were brought into close contact with it.

The technique is to turn in the whole length of the free border of the flap. In the original planning of the flap, allowance must be made for this, in the area that will form the nostrils. It might be expected that two such raw surfaces on the under side of a flap would adhere to each other, but this does not happen as easily as the healing of an incision in the skin. The two surfaces must be brought into close contact, and sutured together. This is best done before the flap is attached, for otherwise there is not enough room, and these sutures may tear out. Both layers are transfixed, as one would stitch a mattress, by a straight needle passing from without inwards, and then from within outwards, so that the knots will lie on the outside. If this heals, the thickened margin of the nostril is much less likely to contract.

PROPORTIONAL STITCHING

This is the term used by tailors for the method of joining a longer edge to a shorter: the short edge is stretched, and the long edge is contracted, avoiding one large fold by making many smaller folds. It is often very useful in plastic surgery. In nearly every flap the free edge is longer than the defect. Each suture must therefore take up a little more of the edge of the flap, so that there is accurate apposition. To ensure that the longer side is made equal to the shorter, the suture nearest to the nostril (in a rhinoplasty), and nearest to the mouth (in a cheiloplasty), must be inserted first. The spacing of the remaining sutures can then be estimated. If they are accurately placed, contraction of the flap will soon even out the edges, however unequal they were at first.

DISPLACEMENT OF SKIN.[28]

Another method discovered by the inexhaustible Dieffenbach, which differs from 'shifting of skin' [transposition],[29] is not designed to construct complete parts, but as a secondary operation to improve their shape. Most reconstructed noses have their greatest prominence in the

[28] [The first description of the V-Y advancement flap.]

[29] See n. 11 above.

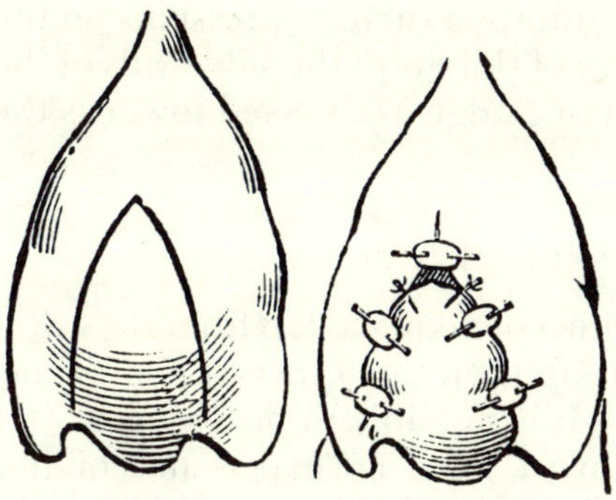

Fig. 13

middle of the bridge, which then falls away sharply, so that the tip does not project. The skin has contracted because of the lack of underlying cartilage, and even if the columella is thick it cannot support the tip.

Two slightly curved incisions are made, meeting at an angle at their upper ends, and forming a flap in the new nose, based below at the columella [Fig. 13]. The upper angle is closed with one twisted suture. This reduces the space for insetting the flap, and proportional stitching must be used. The flap becomes bunched up, making the nose-tip more prominent.

REMOVING EXCESS SKIN FROM THE FLAP

Another technique that is frequently used in secondary operations is the excision of round or oval pieces of skin from a part that is too big. The time to do this is after 6–8 weeks, when all congestion has gone, the skin is no longer shiny, and the little skin creases have reappeared. The excess must not be removed by a horizontal cut, for the wound will granulate, and the patient will be left with a broad scar. The piece of skin to be removed must be calculated beforehand; it is better to make it too small to start with, because more can always be removed later. Incisions are made vertically through the full thickness of the skin down to the underlying tissues, particularly at the angles where the incisions meet; if the under-surface is lying free, as in the nose, this makes a window. The edges of the wound are drawn together to test whether enough skin has been removed. Further narrow strips can then be excised if necessary. After waiting for the bleeding to stop, the wound is closed with twisted sutures.

FILLING SMALL DEFECTS

The same technique can sometimes be used to fill small defects, particularly on the bridge of the nose. If the relation of the diameter of a circle to its circumference is as 1 : 3, the excision of a round piece of skin one inch in diameter will produce a scar one and a half inches long when the wound is undermined and sutured; this pushes the angles of the wound forwards.

Dieffenbach has often used this to improve small depressions on the bridge of the nose, by removing circles of skin from the side walls of the nose, and closing the wounds so that one angle is directed towards the defect.

REPEATED TRANSFER OF A FLAP

Blandin credits Roux with the good idea of taking a flap from the lower lip to reconstruct the cheek, implanting it on the upper lip for a time, and then moving it on.[30] In this way it is possible to provide flaps for parts where there is no skin nearby. I have no experience of this method, but it would seem to offer a reasonable chance of success.[31]

THE PURSE-STRING SUTURE

There is little natural power of healing in a fistula, so that it usually has to be brought about artificially; even this power is counteracted by the discharge through the fistula. Urine is particularly unfavourable, and there is hardly a case known of spontaneous healing of a urinary fistula, either in a man or a woman. After many unsuccessful attempts, using the standard methods, Dieffenbach had the ingenious idea of closing urethral fistulae in men, and vesico-vaginal fistulae in women, by a suture that would narrow the opening concentrically. It is impossible to achieve healing either by encouraging granulations, or by excising the margins and suturing them accurately. But a purse-string suture will bring the margins symmetrically together, even when they are scarred and as hard as cartilage.

A long, strong thread on a curved needle is passed in and out round the opening of the fistula, like the string round a knitting-bag, until the end comes out at the place where it started. When the two ends are pulled tight, and knotted, the opening is symmetrically narrowed, so that it has a chance of healing before the thread cuts out. In a large, scarred fistula, however long the thread remains, it cannot bring about complete and permanent healing. This first suture is intended simply to reduce the size of the opening, and it can be repeated a second, and, if necessary, a third time. If the fistula has been made so small that the margins are in contact, but urine is still leaking through, sutures will have no further effect, and other means must be used to complete the cure—diverting the flow of urine for a time, and stimulating the margins to unite.

---

30 Blandin, *Autoplastie*, p. 162.

31 [See p. 167—case report by Maisonabe.]

LATERAL RELIEVING INCISIONS

On the same principle as Dieffenbach's repeated purse-string sutures to close a fistula, I have made repeated lateral incisions, without suture, to close small holes in the soft palate.[32] These holes are not true fistulae, because they do not lead into a closed and fluid-containing cavity. But they are like fistulae in that their margins are scarred, and healing is delayed by the passage of nasal mucus, saliva, food, and drink; the surrounding tissues are so hard and diseased that concentric healing cannot take place. Closure of small holes in the palate, even when they are enlarged by excising the edges, is impracticable because instruments cannot be introduced into such small openings; touching with caustics (even the famous *tinctura cantharidum concentrata*) will often not produce granulations. However, repeated lateral incisions provide a means of closure by slackening the margins of the opening; while the lateral incisions are healing, the size of the hole is concentrically reduced.

Celsus recommended lateral incisions to relieve tension in the operation for hare-lip.[33] But after his time this important technique was hardly ever used, perhaps for fear of the residual disfigurement or of causing too great an injury. Richter, for example, says: 'these incisions do not help in the hare-lip operation, for they only go through the skin, and it is not this, but the muscle of the lip, that resists stretching; not to mention the disfigurement left by the scars.'[34] As far as I know, it was Dieffenbach who reintroduced this technique into surgery, or at least advised its much wider use. He divides not only the skin, but also the full thickness of the underlying tissues, so that, in a part such as the palate where there are two free surfaces, a window is created. His boldness and his brilliant successes have brought great honour to German surgery.

Plastic operations are, in any case, so painful and traumatic that the addition of two lateral incisions does not greatly increase the injury, in view of the benefit gained; they usually heal with fine linear scars, so that there is little disfigurement. Relieving incisions are particularly useful in forehead rhinoplasty (as well as in the hare-lip operation and reconstruction of the lip), to allow better closure of the defect on the

---

32 [E. Zeis, Heilung eines Loches im weichen Gaumen, welche nach mehren vergeblichen Versuchen der Staphyloraphie zuletzt durch Anlegung von Seitenaperturen ohne Nähte bewirkt ward, *J. Chir. Augenheilk.* **25**, 495 (1837).]

33 See p. 7.

34 A. G. Richter, *Anfangsgründen der Wundarzneikunst*, 3rd edn, Vol. 2 Göttingen, 282 (1802).

forehead. Dieffenbach often makes incisions several inches long on the temples, so that the defect can be closed almost completely. These lateral incisions look terrifying at first, but the central scar becomes almost linear, so that the criticism of the Indian operation—that it leaves a disfiguring scar on the face—can be largely dismissed.

Detailed rules for making relieving incisions cannot be given. In general, the skin should be divided where the tension is greatest. But the incision must not be made too near the wound, so that the bridge between them is not too narrow, and also not too far away, for then there will be little relaxation of the edges of the wound. Relieving incisions have an important part to play in primary healing; this cannot occur if the skin edges have been so forcibly pulled together that their retraction is only prevented by the sutures. The greater the tension, the more the sutures cut out, and this is best prevented by relieving incisions. These are dressed with lint, after careful control of the bleeding, and left to granulate, but they are treated with the same cold compresses as the main wound, to prevent the inflammation becoming too severe. When the central wound has healed, frequent applications of silver nitrate to the exuberant granulations in the lateral incisions will often produce a narrow scar. The relaxation afforded by the lateral incisions is only needed until the main wound has healed; after this, every care must be taken to ensure that they heal as neatly as possible.

DIVISION OF ADHESIONS

In many cases, a deficiency of skin can be made up by dividing its adhesions to the underlying bone. Ulcers of the eyelid adhere to the bone or periosteum because there is little soft tissue between the skin and the bone; it is the same on the forehead. The ulcer causes exfoliation of a piece of the outer table of the bone; this leaves a depressed scar with a very thin layer of tissue over the bone, which cannot be separated from it. If there are scars of this sort, the forehead cannot be used for reconstruction; if the scars are on the sides of the forehead, rhinoplasty can still be carried out, but closure of the wound will be difficult. If the scar is small (and there are not too many of them), an incision can be made round it, leaving it in place, and the skin drawn together over it. If the skin is separated from the bone by muscle and cellular tissue, as in other parts of the face, the adhesion is not as dense as on the forehead, and it is possible to free it; this is urgently needed if the movements of parts of the face, particularly the eyelids and lips, are restricted. The part that has been freed commonly becomes adherent again later, but the tension that this produces does not occur until the main wound has healed soundly; also, the new adhesion is now in a different place.

It is sometimes necessary to divide extensive adhesions of one-third or more of the face. But the reaction to this operation is usually slight, showing that there is little risk to the patient. The rule is to undermine the soft tissues as close to the bone as possible, so that no large vessels or nerves are injured. The half of the face that has been completely separated from the bone retains its normal sensation, and it often recovers more movement than before the operation. A second rule is to prevent, as far as possible, the entry of air into the wound. This is best done by making a small incision some distance away, and separating the tissues through this with a narrow knife. Undermining can also be done through the incision for raising a flap, or, if the adhesions cannot be reached from there, the knife is stabbed in under the upper lip or through the nostril, and all strands are divided by repeated sawing movements until the soft tissues are completely free.

SUTURES

Successful healing in plastic operations depends very largely on the suturing of the flap. The Indian surgeons did not use sutures—at least not in the operation on Cowasjee. Tagliacozzi used simple interrupted sutures; the threads were very long to prevent the ends slipping out before they were tied, and so that there was no need to bring the arm up to the face sooner than necessary. Carpue, in an Indian rhinoplasty, put five sutures in the nose and one in the columella. Such a small number of sutures may be enough if the skin edges fit together exactly. But the application of cold compresses, an involuntary sneeze or cough, or other slight disturbance of the new nose, may destroy the fragile adhesions, if the flap is not held firmly with more sutures. Primary healing will not occur everywhere if there is too great a gap between the sutures.

Gräfe, in the Indian method, used eight sutures in the nose and two in the columella, which were not tied, but closed with ligature-rods.[35] He advised that the lowest sutures should be inserted first. But if these are tied immediately, it is very difficult to pierce the full thickness of the skin with the remaining sutures. Ligature-rods are particularly useful in the Italian and German methods, where there is not enough room between the arm and the head to tie the sutures accurately. The rods allow each suture to be pulled tighter or slackened off as necessary,

[35] Gräfe, *Rhinoplastik*, p. 34.

without having to undo knots. In these two methods, of course, the suturing starts at the upper edge.[36] The disadvantage of the rods is their weight, and Gräfe has recently stopped using them for rhinoplasty. He also recommends that small pieces of ivory or boxwood should be put under the sutures, if the skin edges overlap as they are tightened.[37] Each piece is somewhat convex on the side which is laid on the edge of the wound, and flat on the other, with a small notch to hold the suture. This is somewhat similar to the old quilled suture, where a long quill is laid on each side of the wound, and the threads are knotted over them; the quills do not cover the wound, but they exert even pressure on the gaps between the sutures. Gräfe's small plaques, however, are laid directly on the wound to bring the edges into exact apposition without overlapping, and the threads are tied over them to hold them in place. I have no personal experience of them, but it seems that their small size, as shown in Gräfe's illustration [Fig. 14], means that they could easily be pushed into the wound, with very harmful results. Most plastic surgeons now do not use them.

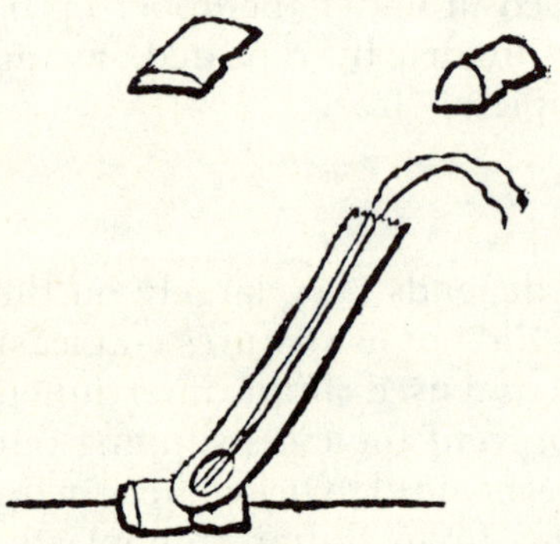

Fig. 14

Interrupted sutures tend to make the skin edges overlap or invert (inversion occurs particularly when there is no firm base under the wound); they have been superseded by Dieffenbach's twisted sutures.

The twisted suture

This is the old hare-lip suture, modified by Dieffenbach, and first used by him for rhinoplasty; it is commonly known as Dieffenbach's suture.[38] Moderately fine Carlsbad insect-pins are inserted (like the needles for interrupted sutures) 1–2 lines from the edge of the wound,[39] through the full thickness of the skin, taking care that the exit on the opposite side is symmetrical with the insertion—not further away from the edge, nor more superficial. The pin is pushed by its head through to its midpoint,

[36] Ibid. p. 142.

[37] Ibid. p. 35.

[38] J. F. Dieffenbach, 'Die abgeänderte umschlungene Nath als schnelles Heilmittel bei Gesichtswunden', *Annln. ges. Heilk.* **8**, 129 (1827).

[39] [One line = 1/12 inch.]

and the protruding ends are wrapped round 5–6 times, as in the well-known hare-lip suture, with circular and figure-of-eight turns of thick unwaxed cotton. This is knotted, and the projecting ends of the pin are cut off. The ends of the thread are used to pull up the edges of the wound, to make the insertion of the next pin easier, and they are then cut near the knot. In most cases it is not necessary to put the sutures closer than 3–5 lines apart, for the twisting of the thread pulls the edges together in the gaps between the sutures, and only a very narrow strip of skin remains uncovered.

The pins are removed by pulling with forceps on the end furthest from the flap, to avoid pulling the flap away from its new bed. If the end of the pin was cut cleanly, so that it is not bent, removal is usually easy. The twisted thread falls off on its own, or is easily lifted off. There is usually a little bleeding from the stitch-holes on both sides, which relieves the irritation of removing the pins. Sometimes the pin is held by dried blood, so that it must be gently turned in its long axis before it can be removed. If it cannot be removed because the end is bent, either this is cut off again, or the thread is cut through or unwound.

The advantages of Dieffenbach's sutures are so great that, whenever they can be used, they are preferred above all others. The suturing of divided muscles has now been almost abandoned, and sutures are used mostly only for the skin. If it is ever thought to be necessary to join deeper structures, interrupted sutures are better. In the skin, however, there is only one situation where twisted sutures cannot be used—where two edges have to be joined in a deep angle, e,g. where the columella is set into the upper lip, or at the inner canthus of the eye. Sometimes even this can be achieved by bending the pin, before it is inserted, into the same curve as the needle for interrupted sutures. But the ends may still irritate the skin, even when they have been cut as short as possible. In such cases, simple interrupted sutures should be used, but they should be put close together, to give some of the advantages of twisted sutures.

Twisted sutures should be used for all facial wounds, and when a very fine scar is desirable. They are an essential part of plastic surgery, which would never have achieved so much without them. With interrupted sutures, the skin edges are not accurately apposed in the gaps between the sutures. Sticking-plaster helps a little, but less so in plastic operations where only very short strips can be used, which soon slacken or fall off. With twisted sutures the cotton thread absorbs blood and serum, and this increases the area of apposition. It also protects the wound from the air, so that it is not necessary to use dressings, which interfere with the application of cold compresses. The smooth surface of the pin (made of tin-plated brass wire) produces no harmful chemical reaction, and it seems to provoke even less reaction than silk or linen. The cotton thread only comes in contact with the epidermal surface of the skin, so that there is no need to use anything more compatible with the tissues; linen and silk tend to cut in more, and they absorb less fluid. When many twisted sutures are inserted close together, the edges of the wound are lifted up like a seam. This does not matter, for as soon as the pins are removed the edges sink back to the level of the surrounding skin. The pressure of the twisted threads makes the edges of the wound pale, by keeping the blood out of them. But this encourages healing (as long as they are not too tight), for congestion of the edges of a wound quickly leads to suppuration.

11

NOSE—RHINOPLASTY[1]

RECONSTRUCTION OF THE WHOLE NOSE

The nose can be reconstructed in whole or in part. The former is much less common, although carcinoma, or syphilis (especially if this has been treated homoeopathically for a long time), can sometimes destroy the whole nose, so that no trace of the bone remains. In many cases the bone has been attacked, but it has only sunk in a little, because it is supported by the septum, or because only part of the bone has been extruded. Most commonly the tip of the nose and the anterior halves of the alae are missing. Wounds always remove only the anterior cartilaginous part, for if the cut goes deeper it is usually incomplete, and the part can be reattached so that no plastic operation is needed. Even *herpes exedens nasi* stops when it has destroyed the anterior part of the nose.[2] If the whole nose is missing, leaving a large hole, the vomer and turbinates have usually also been destroyed, particularly in syphilis, although they are often retained in carcinoma. True cancer is rarely curable, even if its ulcerated surface has been completely scarred over by silver nitrate or similar means. The advanced age at which this disease mostly occurs, and its malignancy, make the prognosis very uncertain, and it is always the most unfavourable indication for rhinoplasty.

Not only does loss of the whole nose indicate more severe and long-standing disease, but reconstruction is more difficult, needing a very large flap. Even if the rotated pedicle, in the Indian method, gives a better restoration of the root of the nose, the Italian method may be preferable if the forehead cannot provide enough skin. Bünger, in such circumstances, decided to use a piece of skin completely detached from the thigh.[3] But an experienced surgeon knows how much he can take from the forehead, and how the defect that this leaves may seem enormous, but that it causes little reaction, and does not leave a very disfiguring scar. There is no general rule, and each surgeon must

---

[1] *Rhin,* the nose, and *plassein,* to form.

[2] [See p. 53, n, 1.]

[3] See p. 21, n, 20.

choose for himself which method to use. But it must be said that the Italian operation is more difficult, with many more chances of failure, and it depends too much for its success on the co-operation of the patient. No surgeon doing a rhinoplasty for the first time should choose Tagliacozzi's or Gräfe's methods.

Tagliacozzi does not state clearly whether he ever did a total rhinoplasty. His book contains no case histories, and the illustrations only show deformities of the nose with the lower part missing. Carpue's and Gräfe's cases are the same. Dieffenbach was the first to undertake reconstruction of the whole nose. He always tries to conserve as much as possible of the remnants of the old nose, and he limits the reconstruction to the actual loss of tissue. But when the whole nose has to be replaced, he is, as always, the boldest plastic surgeon of them all.

It is not my intention in this book to describe every operation in detail. Every plastic surgical case varies, and each surgeon must use his own judgement. I have already said enough about the general technique of rhinoplasty in previous chapters, so that here it is only necessary to describe the main variations from the standard operation. The flap for a total reconstruction must have a broader pedicle than that needed simply to nourish a flap for the lower half, for the pedicle will form the upper part of the nose. This makes rotation of the flap more difficult, but this can be overcome by wide undermining, and by extending one of the incisions down to the defect.[4]

When there is no nose, the incisions to receive the flap must be made in the skin of the face at the margins of the defect. Experience rather than exact measurement will tell the surgeon how far from the defect to make them, to prevent the new nose having too broad a base and being too flat. The junction of skin and mucous membrane is often scarred, and it is better to avoid it. This is not always possible in such large defects, and the flap must be inserted into scar-tissue; in my experience this usually heals quite well. Suturing is difficult in such indurated tissues; the insect-pins often bend, so that they have to be removed, and new ones inserted.

Von Ammon's case of total reconstruction

In 1834 I watched von Ammon operate for total loss of the nose. The patient was a jobbing gardener who had had an ulcer of his nose for 5–6 years. This was thought to be cancer, and was treated homoeopathically, although it was undoubtedly syphilitic, as shown by its

[4] See p. 87.

dramatic cure by inunctions [of mercury]. When it was completely healed he came under von Ammon's care with total loss of the nose. Other deformities of his face needed eight major operations to give him a more human appearance; several of these were carried out to allow him to open his mouth, by separating adhesions of his cheeks to his jaw, caused by the over-use of mercury. A preliminary attempt was made to reconstruct the columella from the upper lip (to make the subsequent rhinoplasty easier, as the forehead was rather low), but it was destroyed by gangrene. On 4 March, von Ammon raised a flap on the forehead, which included some hairy scalp for the columella and part of the alae. After the flap had been brought down into place, the wound in the forehead was sutured at its upper and lower ends, with a relieving incision in one temple. Because of the scarring on the face the pedicle was made very broad, so that wide undermining was needed to allow it to rotate without tension. Parts of the skin of the face were so scarred that it was impossible to insert the pins for twisted sutures, and interrupted sutures had to be used.[5] This patient was one of those who suffered unbearable photophobia immediately after the flap was raised; in this case, however, it continued after the end of the operation, and it was still troublesome on the third day.[6] On the fifth day after operation the patient could smell again, which he had not been able to do for a long time. The flap healed well, but part of the columella was lost, and had to be replaced later—again from the upper lip.

Repeated operations

People used to run away from the patient described above, because of his hideous deformity, so that he could not join in the communal work in the fields, but had to work by himself. His concern over his appearance, and his burning desire to return to human company, gave him the courage to withstand not only the rhinoplasty, but also the other major operations, with amazing fortitude. But in the end he showed what is so commonly seen—that the bravest and apparently most insensitive patients finally become cowardly and fearful of the knife after repeated operations. He bore eight very painful operations, and only cried out at the last, and was as frightened as a child

[5] This experience made von Ammon turn, in later cases, to English sewing-needles as sharper and less flexible. But they have the disadvantage that, after 24–48 hours in the tissues, the steel becomes so oxidized that they can only be removed with great difficulty—perhaps this could be avoided by having them gold-plated.

[6] [See p. 76.]

beforehand. Although this often happens, Labat and Blandin are to be criticized for advising against secondary plastic operations on the grounds that patients cannot summon the resolution necessary to submit to them, once they have withstood the original operation.[7] For it is not as bad as that. Even if the patients become more frightened and more sensitive with each operation, they will still gladly undergo secondary operations, if they can be assured that these are quite slight (compared with the original), and that the shape of the new nose is going to be much improved.

Dieffenbach's principle

This advice by Labat and Blandin is quite contrary to the principle on which Dieffenbach works, and which, as experience has shown, is undoubtedly correct. According to him, all measurements and calculations of how big the new nose should be are useless, and the attempt to make it perfect at the first operation only results in it being too small. It cannot be stressed enough, to those who have no experience of plastic operations, that the best nose is one that, immediately after the operation (and even more in the next few days when it is swollen and congested), looks an over-sized shapeless lump. When all this has subsided, and the flap is still too big, it can be reduced; this will cause the patient very little pain. Only tissue that is then really in excess is removed, and this cannot be estimated before the flap has contracted.

RECONSTRUCTION OF THE LOWER PART OF THE NOSE

Most cases coming to reconstruction have lost only the lower (cartilaginous) part of the nose. Parts of the alae and columella remain, which can be used, and the flap must be modified accordingly. The Indian operation is the commonest, and might be called the 'normal' operation. For most cases, the outer of the two patterns [Fig. 15] is more suitable, assuming that the defect is symmetrical. The edges *ab*, *ba* will be sutured to the lateral edges of the defect; *bc* and *cb* will be the free borders of the alae and the columella. The dotted line *cc* is the part of the columella to be joined to the upper lip, but it is better to cut it to a point *d*; this makes it easier to close this part of the defect in the forehead. The patient, who has more than enough to put up with, is spared a little pain if the triangle *cdc* is excised after the flap has been raised, while it is still relatively insensitive.

---

[7] See p. 87.

The inner pattern is Gräfe's model for the Indian method; it differs mainly in its smaller size and the narrowness of the columella. But the columella can never be too broad, to allow for contraction; one of this size will always be too thin. It is the same with the whole flap—it can never be too big. The shape of the defect and the thickness of the skin will also determine the shape of the flap.

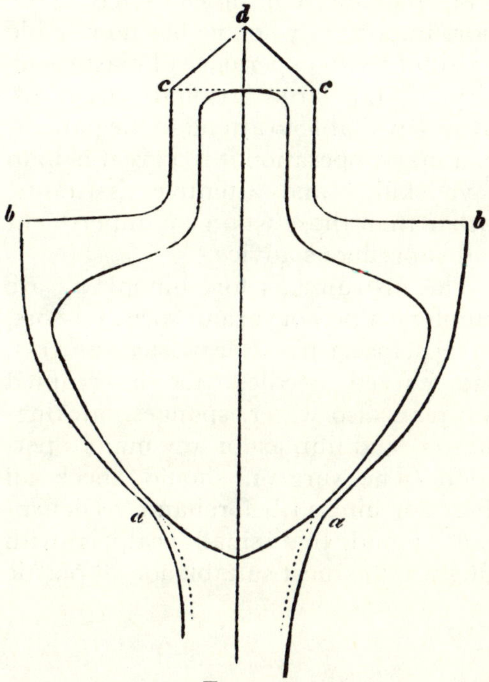

Fig. 15

Delpech[8] raises a flap with three long points, so that the forehead wound is easier to close. The tips are cut off, as shown by the dotted lines [Fig. 16]. But this flap is too small for a complete reconstruction, and it can only be used, as in his patient, for the tip of the nose. Dieffenbach has recently used an oval flap [Fig. 17]. Two cuts are made with scissors to form the columella and the alae; the former is sutured to the upper lip, and the oblique ends of the latter are turned in and held in place with sutures. This method is useful with very thin skin, for it gives the tip greater stability, and prevents contraction of the nostrils. Labat is said to have raised a similar flap, which is broader and more rounded. If the skin is thick, Dieffenbach finds that an oval flap is impractical, because the edges are either too thick to be turned in, or they make the margins of the nostrils too thick.

Pre-operative preparation

When it is certain that there is no underlying disease, when the patient's affairs have been so arranged that he is relaxed and looking forward to his new life, and when he is in as cheerful a frame of mind as anyone awaiting a painful operation, then the day and the hour of the

[8] Delpech, *Chirurgie clinique*, Vol. 2, p. 225 (1828).

operation can be fixed. But he must not be told this. Even the most courageous patient should be left in ignorance until the last minute.

There is still one thing to be considered—the surgeon himself. Not only does the operation take time, but the after-treatment demands the greatest care and attention. The operation may have to be postponed because the surgeon's time is taken up with too many other patients, as in an epidemic. This precaution is all the more important when he has no reliable assistants with experience of plastic surgery; in the large hospitals these are always available to attend to the patient. In a major operation it is a great help to have skilled and attentive assistants, rather than those who give impertinent and superfluous advice.[9]

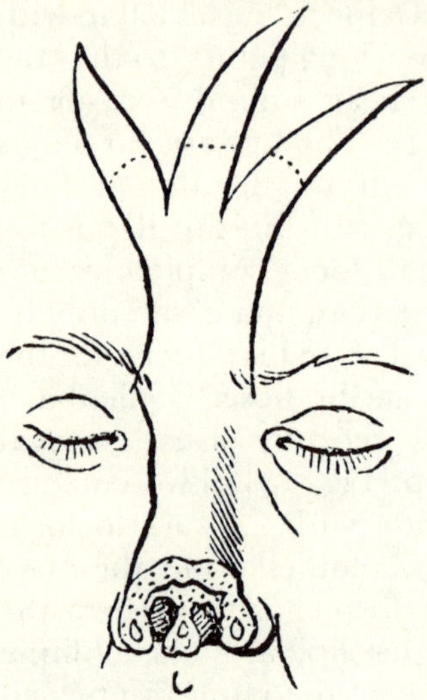

Fig. 16

The instruments for rhinoplasty are simple: scalpels of various sorts, scissors, forceps, insect-pins (for twisted sutures), and curved needles (for interrupted sutures); also water, sponges, sticking-plaster, and lint, as for any major operation. The surgeon should check all these for himself beforehand.[10] Dieffenbach found that small scalpels with octagonal cataract-needle handles are the most suitable for all plastic operations.

Now, to work!

Operative technique

The patient sits on a stool facing the window; if he is lying down, blood will run into his throat and make him cough. Once the size and shape of the flap have been decided, the pattern is cut out of paper or sticking-plaster. The outline of a paper pattern is marked on the forehead with dye, but this is quickly obliterated by blood at the start of the operation. It is better to

[9] 'The attendants must observe diligently every nod of the surgeon, for many things happen during an operation which need to be indicated by a nod, and not by speech, One must be sparing of words on account of the patient.' Tagliacozzi, *de curtorum*, Vol. 2, Chapter 4, p. 12.

[10] 'For nothing will be done that you do not do yourself, It is an important part of the task to be sufficiently provided with suitable instruments, and to have them prepared and laid out in advance. This gives the surgeon an additional advantage, enhancing both the art and the artist.' Tagliacozzi, *de curtorum*, Vol. 2, Chapter 7. p. 23.

cut the pattern in plaster, and to stick this to the forehead; it is removed when the flap has been raised. But the plaster must be of the best quality, which comes away cleanly, and does not make the skin sticky.

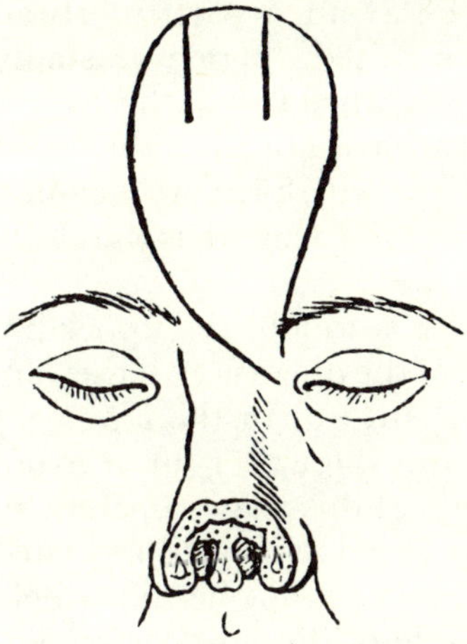

Fig. 17

The operation starts with excision of the margins of the remnants of the nose. Gräfe recommends that the skin should be incised first, then the mucosa, and then the intervening strip removed, where it is adherent to the cartilage; but a single incision through the full thickness gives much cleaner edges. Then the incision for the attachment of the columella is made in the upper lip: the lip is pulled hard away from the upper jaw, and pierced with a scalpel, where it joins the jaw, in full thickness for one inch, or a little more if the columella is broader. This may seem excessive, but if the incision is not deep enough the columella will not unite, especially as interrupted, and not twisted, sutures have to be used.

The flap is raised from the forehead by inserting a bistoury at right angles to the skin at the upper end, and carrying the incision down round each side of the pattern through the full thickness of the skin. On one side the incision extends to between the eyebrows, and, on the other, along the bridge of the nose down to the defect. With a hooked forceps in the left hand (better than the ordinary toothed forceps, as it does not slip), the flap is undermined, starting at the upper end. The assistants must keep the wound clean by dabbing with a soft sponge, for there is the danger of damaging the galea, which must be preserved, or of stripping too much underlying tissue off the flap, or even making a hole in it. When the flap has been freed down to its pedicle, the triangle *cdc* at the tip of the columella is excised (see Fig. 15). The flap is rotated down so that its epidermal surface is on the outside, and tested to see that it will lie comfortably in the defect. If there is any tension, the pedicle is further undermined, and the incision round the flap is extended down a little. It is essential that one end of the incision reaches the defect. This not only makes the rotation easier, but reduces the size of the swelling caused by the rotated pedicle, and, most important, provides a larger attachment for the flap.[11]

[11] [See p. 87.]

The greatest care is now taken to stop the bleeding, for there is no hurry to suture the flap, and it is even an advantage to wait.[12] A dressing is put on the forehead, and fixed with sticking-plaster to prevent contact with the air, which is to be avoided particularly in wounds of the head. After the flap has been raised, there are usually several spurting arteries, most often at the glabella, but this is not serious. It is easy to catch and twist them; ligation is not advisable, even with very fine thread, for this would interfere with primary healing. When the bleeding has completely stopped, the wound is carefully cleaned before suturing.

Suturing should start where the columella is to join the upper lip, using long threads which are tied at the end of the operation; if they are tied immediately, it makes the insertion of sutures in the alae very difficult. Three or four threads are inserted in the upper lip; it is not necessary to pass them through the columella at this stage, for this can easily be done later. The rest of the flap is attached with twisted sutures. It must be emphasized that these should not be too widely spaced; three interrupted sutures in each side of the nose, as recommended by Beck,[13] are not enough. Healing by first intention can only occur if the edges of the wound are in the closest apposition; increasing the number of sutures only increases the reaction very slightly. If there is too wide a space between two sutures, a finer insect-pin or an interrupted suture should be inserted. The defect in the forehead can be closed with twisted sutures near the glabella and in the part from which the columella came. A gap in the centre of less than one or one and a half inches can be sutured after relieving incisions in the temples, but a gap larger than this must be left to heal by granulation. The forehead and lateral incisions are dressed with lint and strips of sticking-plaster. With twisted sutures, plaster is unnecessary on the nose.

Post-operative care

The patient has for a long time been accustomed to the free passage of air through the nasal defect, so that now, to avoid him having to breathe through his mouth all the time, little tubes, which will not collapse, are placed in the new nostrils. These were usually pieces of quill, covered with linen, and greased. I have recently been making them out of the discs of indiarubber, which are now being produced commercially, and which should have many other uses in surgery. The

---

[12] [See p. 18.]

[13] C. J. Beck, Gelungener Fall einer Rhinoplastik, *Heidelb. klin. Annln.* **3,** 250 (1827).

material is soft, so that there is no need to cover it. Tubes can very quickly be made to fit in all shapes and sizes, so that they do not fall out. They are changed every few days, taking care, if they are sticky with dried mucus, that their removal does not disrupt the newly adherent tissues. When rubber has been in the nose too long it becomes white and soft; but as soon as it is dry it regains its old properties, and it can be used again.

If, on the day of the operation and the next day, the new nose is flat (see Plate 1 (a)), and bears not the faintest resemblance to a nose, there should be no anxiety that the flap will not swell. Often the swelling develops only too quickly and excessively; the skin-folds disappear, and the flap becomes shiny and light red, and then dark red and blueish. The full anti-inflammatory regime must be started, to keep the inflammation at the low level necessary for primary healing.[14]

The pins of the twisted sutures are removed on the third or fourth day. The thread is then easily lifted off, and the stitch-holes are allowed to bleed dry; if union is uncertain, small strips of English plaster are laid across the scar.[15]

Dieffenbach's first case

In 1828 I had the opportunity to see and admire Dieffenbach's first case of reconstruction of the lower part of the nose. The patient was a healthy young man who had come home safely after many adventures by land and sea, but then lost his nose in a duel. An attempt had been made to reattach it, but it went gangrenous. The wound soon healed, and he wore a nose of laquered silver. But he found this irksome, and he made himself a nose-tip out of red English plaster, which he changed every day. He came to Dieffenbach in Berlin asking for reconstruction.[16]

The first step in the operation was to raise a narrow strip, based above, from each alar margin, turning it over so that its epidermal surface was on the inside, and suturing it to the freshened upper border of the septum. This was an attempt to raise the height of the septum and increase the prominence of the bridge of the nose; with such a small attachment it was doubtful whether union between the strips of skin and the cartilage would occur. Then a pear-shaped flap was raised from the centre of the forehead, carrying the incisions down on both

[14] [See p. 70.]

[15] ['Court' plaster, as used by fashionable ladies for decorative patches on the face.]

[16] Dieffenbach, *Erfahrungen,* Vol. 2 p. 38 (1830).

sides of the root of the nose. The flap was sutured into the defect with 12 insect-pins; two more sutures fixed the flap to the septum, and four stronger sutures were placed in the forehead, which was under great tension.

The patient showed exemplary courage and endurance, and scarcely made a sound. Because he was unusually strong and healthy, he was at once put on a strict anti-inflammatory diet of thin gruel and lemonade, and his bowels were kept open with Epsom salts. His forehead was covered with ice-packs, and his nose with wet dressings. In spite of all these precautions, as well as massive blood-letting and the repeated application of leeches, such severe inflammation of the nose and cheeks developed that it was feared that the flap would go gangrenous.

It is interesting to record the colour changes in the flap: immediately it had been freed from the forehead it became blueish; 6–8 minutes later it was pale in the middle and dark blue at the margins. After it had been sutured it was bright red and a little swollen. As the pedicle was rather broad, and therefore too sharply compressed, its most prominent point was excised obliquely. At once an artery started spurting, and the flap became pale and collapsed; the bleeding was allowed to continue at a slower rate for several hours. Eight hours after the operation the flap was light-red, somewhat swollen, and with a normal temperature. The next morning there was marked swelling, redness, and warmth, which increased towards evening. Eight pins were removed, and lukewarm water was applied to encourage the stitch-holes to bleed for several hours. On the fourth day all the remaining sutures were removed, and the wound was soundly healed. The swelling began to subside, and by the eighth day all parts of the face had returned to normal, except the tip of the nose. Here the skin was dry and shiny, and it desquamated over the next few days. At two weeks, the pedicle formed a hump on the bridge of the nose, and it seemed that this was the time to excise it, together with the part that had been inset into the bridge. But the patient refused, because he was still afraid that the flap might die. After five weeks they were excised, and the original skin edges were reunited with four insect-pins; with the application of cold dressings this wound healed in five days. The patient was delighted with his appearance, and Dieffenbach showed him to other surgeons, and to many doctors at a medical meeting, who all praised the result. Although the tip of the nose was perhaps not long enough, the bridge was a good height, giving him a somewhat aquiline, English profile. The colour was the same as the rest of his face, and the scars on his forehead and nose were hardly visible.

When Dieffenbach saw him seven years later, his nose had not

(a)

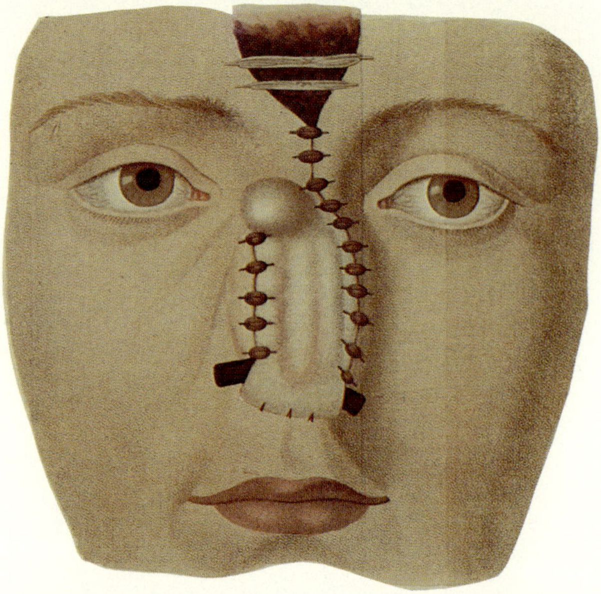

(b)

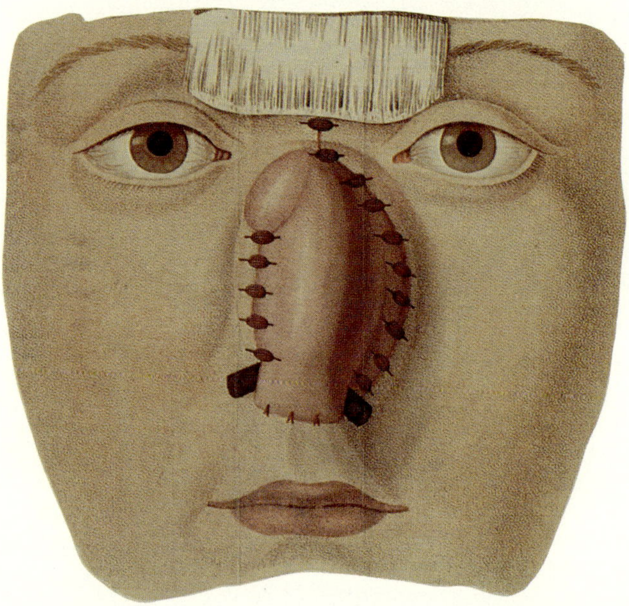

Pl. 1. (a) A nose, reconstructed from the forehead, immediately after the operation. The flap has hardly changed colour; this shows that the operation should be successful. Even in this view from the front it can be seen that the nose is lying quite flat. The flap is so slack that it moves with every breath. Dieffenbach's twisted sutures have been used for the greater part of the flap, with interrupted sutures for the columella. There are small rubber tubes in the nostrils. (b) The same, the next day. The nose now projects well forward. The colour has altered as the flap has become more congested. The shininess and stretching of the skin at this stage are not easy to show in a drawing. This degree of activity in the flap needs the most vigorous application of cold compresses. If the congestion increases any further, local blood-letting will be essential.

(a)

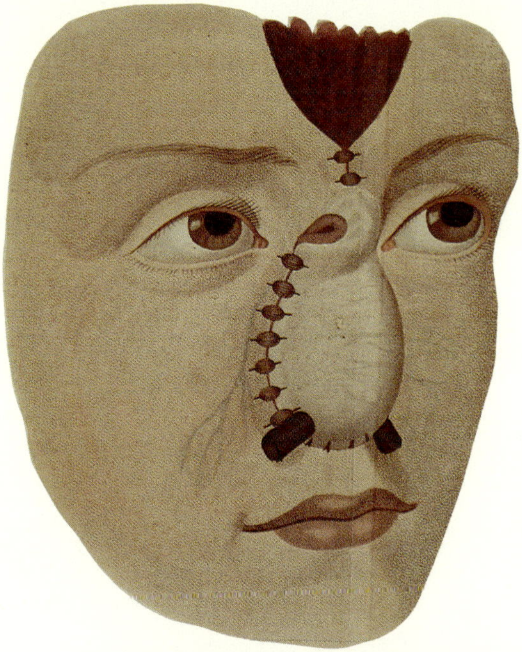

(b)

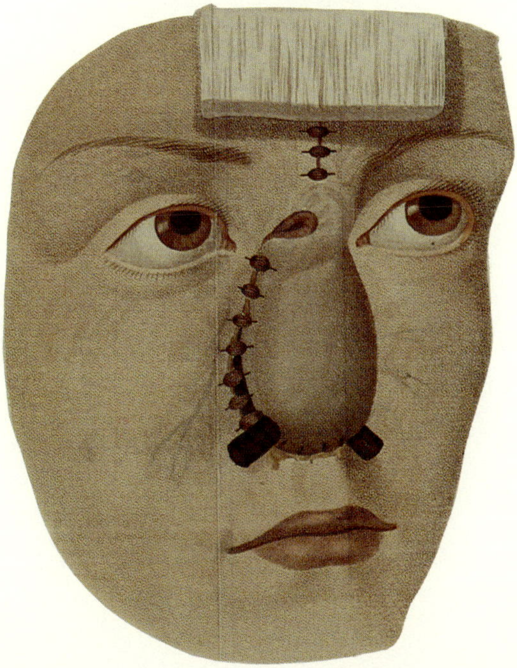

Pl. 2. (a) A reconstructed nose on the second day, which already looks likely to die. The flap is swollen, but the skin itself is not as robust as in Plate 1., so that small creases can be seen in it. There is a network of scars on the face, and also on the pedicle, which is interfering with the blood-supply. It is paler than the rest of the face. The edges of the wound have not united, and it is only held together by the sutures. (b) The same, the next day. All is as good as lost. There is no union, and pus is pouring out. A narrow strip on the right side has been destroyed by dry gangrene. The rest of the nose is a sinister blue colour, so that it will soon go the same way.

altered. The favourable factors in this case were the excellent health of the patient, and the fact that the defect was caused by external injury. Against these was the extreme irritability of his skin, with a strong tendency to erysipelas; even the application of sticking-plaster caused inflammation. Without strenuous anti-inflammatory measures, the operation might have been a failure. Dieffenbach felt some anxiety about this case, as it was the first time that he had transplanted a piece of the forehead to the tip of the nose. There was also the question of the incision of the normal skin on the bridge of the nose for insetting the pedicle; if the flap had become gangrenous, or the pedicle infected, the undermining of the skin and exposure of the nasal bones could have resulted in destruction of the bridge of the nose. With further experience of the operation, Dieffenbach blamed himself, in this case, for making the flap too short, and the pedicle too broad.

Labat's modification

It is not possible to describe all the minor variations which different surgeons have introduced in individual cases of rhinoplasty. But there is one that Labat uses to make the alae unite more easily, and to prevent a prominent scar on the side of the nose.[17] The incision round the flap is not perpendicular to the skin, but, in the lower two-thirds, obliquely outwards, and in the upper third, obliquely inwards, leaving less epidermis on the skin that is to form the alae, and more on the skin for the free border of the nostrils. This means that the former will project more when they are sutured, while the latter can be turned in more easily. The preparation of the defect is made with corresponding oblique incisions, i.e. outwards in the upper part, and inwards in the lower. It is doubtful whether there is much advantage in this, for one cannot forecast if a scar will be prominent, and, if this happens, it can be excised more easily than one that is depressed.

The use of hair-bearing skin

Dieffenbach believes that hairy scalp can be used to make a nose when there is not enough local tissue in the defect, and when the raising of a very large flap would leave too big a scar on the forehead. One advantage is the greater thickness of the scalp, which often has an almost cartilaginous texture. But the question is whether a flap from such a distance can be nourished through a narrow pedicle, and, also,

[17] Labat, *De la rhinoplastie*, p. 68.

how to deal with the growth of hair. Noses made from the arm sometimes have a luxuriant growth of hair, so that it seems likely that the scalp will do the same. Dieffenbach assumed that skin with a high vitality, when reduced to a lower vitality by transplantation, would grow hair, but that skin of a low vitality, transplanted to a bed with a higher vitality, would become acclimatized, and would lose its hair. This is indeed what happens, but there is a more likely explanation: the fine hairs of the arm have their roots in the dermis, while the thicker scalp hairs have their roots in the tissue deep to the dermis, and thus they are exposed when a flap is raised; they are further deprived of nourishment when the under-surface of the flap becomes scarred, so that they either fall out or can be easily plucked out. After Dieffenbach had experimented by making a columella out of hairy skin,[18] he proceeded to reconstruct three noses from the scalp.[19] At the present time he will only use the scalp when the forehead is too scarred. Exposure of the skull makes this more dangerous than using the forehead.

USING THE REMAINS OF THE OLD NOSE

Any healthy parts of the old nose should be retained; the standard pattern for the flap is altered to accommodate them. In one of my cases I was able to build up the right side of the nose from a sunken piece of skin that remained.

Case-report A girl of sixteen, after many years of inflammation of the eyes, which left her with a corneal opacity, developed ulceration of her nose. After much fruitless treatment, her mother confessed to the doctor that she had had syphilitic ulceration of the genitalia during the pregnancy and at the time of the girl's birth. Specific treatment of the girl, especially with gold, then healed the ulcers, but her nose had been destroyed. She was left with a large hole in the centre of her face in which the bones were exposed, giving her the appearance of a skull with eyes. All that remained was part of the skin of the bridge of the nose, and this was deeply sunken in. However, she was extremely vain, dressing herself up with huge ear-rings, and always smiling, which made her look more hideous than ever. As a result of destruction of the internal bones of her nose she was very deaf, so that you had to come very close if you wanted to speak to her, and it was then impossible to avoid being blasted by the stinking breath coming out of this great hole.

---

[18] Dieffenbach, *Erfahrungen,* Vol. 2, p. 52 (1830).

[19] Ibid. pp. 85, 90, 100.

She was longing for the operation, but I wanted to wait and see whether the exposed bone would be extruded, as it would have been very difficult to remove it later through the nostrils. However, there was no sign of natural sequestration, and I thought that there was no need to wait any longer. I decided to carry out a preliminary operation to test her healing power, for, although the ulcers had been cured, the skin of her forehead was very thin, and she was generally sickly, with irregular menstruation, and occasionally coughing up blood.

On 9 November 1836 I freed the sunken piece of skin, unrolling it by light incisions on its inner surface, and attached it to the stump of the right ala with four twisted sutures, to form one side-wall of the nose. This healed by first intention. On 25 November I carried out the reconstruction with a forehead flap, shaped as in Fig. 18. The columella came from hairy skin that had been shaved beforehand. The patient could feel the prick of the needles in the flap, but she had little sensation of touch. The flap at first hung slackly, moving with every breath, so that no-one would have taken it for a nose. But it soon started to swell, and by the third day it was projecting nicely; its colour was a little redder than the rest of the face. The columella failed to unite with the upper lip, but the rest of the flap healed well, although the right side tended to return to its original site, pulling the nose over.

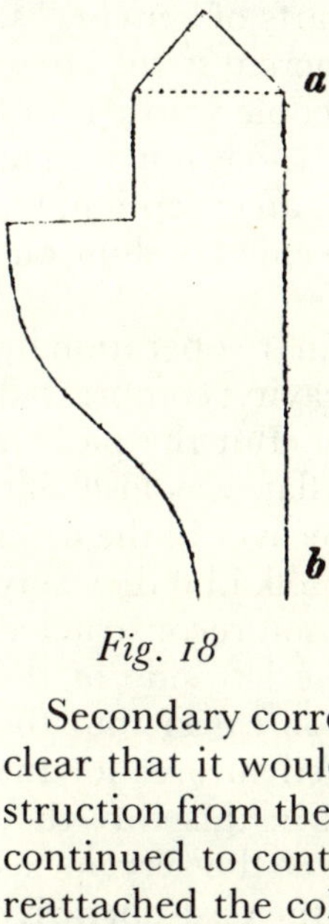

Fig. 18

Secondary correction was carried out on 18 December, but it became clear that it would have been better to have made a complete reconstruction from the forehead, without retaining the original parts, which continued to contract and distort the new nose. On 5 January 1837 I reattached the columella to the upper lip; although it was at least an inch wide at first, it had contracted into the rounded shape of a normal columella. Although the girl has withstood so many painful operations, and has been left with a tolerable appearance (which could be improved by further secondary operations), she has developed phthisis, and it seems likely that this will soon end her life.

INCREASING THE SIZE OF A RECONSTRUCTED NOSE WITH A SECOND FLAP

When a flap from the forehead has contracted so much that the nose does not match the face, and if the patient is willing, the operation can be repeated. The following case of von Ammon's is the only example so far.

Case report A healthy peasant-girl aged 17 had, four years before, suffered from ulcers which destroyed her nose, and left her with multiple scars on her face and in many parts of her body. She had been healed for two years. The cause was uncertain, but the pattern of scars on her face made syphilis the most likely—possibly complicated by some sort of scrofula. The wonder was that the disease had been so completely cured. Her nose had collapsed, but part of the bone was still present, and she could breathe through a small scarred hole. A network of shiny scars, with small reddish vessels, covered parts of her cheeks, and extended up to the left upper eyelid; this was adherent to the bone, as a result of caries, but without ectropion. Most people whose noses have been destroyed look so appalling that someone who is not used to the sight regards them as evil-doers. But this girl was an exception, for she had such beautiful blue eyes that her innocence seemed to shine out of them, and the loss of her nose was almost forgotten.

On 10 May 1836 von Ammon carried out a preliminary operation by making a columella out of the skin closing the nasal cavity; compressed sponge was placed in the nasal opening to dilate it. But the patient developed erysipelas of the face and scalp, and the flap was lost. She was sent home for several weeks, so that she could recover in the fresh air, for the lack of this will sometimes make country folk ill if they stay any length of time in the city. On 27 June von Ammon reconstructed the nose. The flap had to be taken more from the left side of the forehead, because of scarring; this made the rotation easier, but the pedicle was close to a scarred area. Four interrupted sutures for the columella were inserted first, but not pulled tight; in this way they could be inserted very accurately. There was anxiety that erysipelas would again ruin the result, particularly as many of the post-operative patients at that time were suffering from it, but luckily this did not occur. Over the next few days the patient hardly complained, and the flap remained a good colour; when it was touched, she felt the sensation in the new site and not in her forehead. The nostrils were held open with rubber tubes. By the fifth day all sutures had been removed, and the flap had healed well. The nose was still rather flat, partly because the flap was too narrow, and partly because the columella had been set too low. The forehead produced laudable pus, but by 17 July it had not completely healed, and the patient was sent home again.

She came back six weeks later looking very well, but her nose was too small. She was quite willing to have another operation if it would bring further improvement. On 17 September, therefore, von Ammon split the nose down the middle, and filled the defect with a flap from the right side of the forehead. This pedicle came to lie in the same place as the first one, making a sizeable hummock. The right side healed with a linear scar, but there was suppuration on the left, resulting in a depressed scar. The original flap thus formed the side-walls of the nose, and the second flap formed the bridge. This is certainly the largest nose that has ever been constructed. Unfortunately it has the faults of nearly all the new noses so far. The columella, in spite of its size, is not able to support the tip of the nose. But even if it could do this, there is never enough tissue to make the tip project like a normal nose. The greatest height is in the middle, and the tip curves down from there, instead of standing out at an angle. The nostrils contract, however large they are made to start with, and they come to serve more for appearance than for breathing.

On 21 October von Ammon made a flap of the excess skin from the two pedicles, which he transplanted into the tip of the nose; he also excised the depressed scar on the left side. Unfortunately this was followed by gangrene which destroyed part of the new flap, as well as a strip along the scar. In cases like this, healing will eventually occur by secondary intention, but the scar is never as good as when it heals primarily. Even if the scar is not broad, it will always leave a groove that disfigures the nose, betraying the fact that this was created by human hand. This all shows how much we rely on the power of Nature, and how the plastic surgeon must never give up his work for lost, even if the reconstructed part has turned out to be too small. But it is certainly much more difficult to correct this than to reduce a part that is too big—if this should ever happen!

THE INSERTION OF METAL SUPPORTS FOR THE NOSE

Rust,[20] Klein,[21] and Galenzowsky[22] have tried to support collapsed noses by inserting gold discs, and Klein reported that he had corrected a man's saddle-nose with a gold plate. Tyrrell, surgeon at St. Thomas's

[20] J. N. Rust, Neue Methode verstümmelte und durchbrochene Nasen auszubessern. Ein Beitrag zur Geschichte der Nasenrestaurationen, *Magazin. ges, Heilk.* **2** 351 (1817).

[21] K. C. von Klein, Hingeworfene chirurg. Bruchstücke, *Heidelb. klin. Anniln.* **2,** 103 (1826).

[22] In R. Sick, Ueber einige durch Armhautüberpflanzungen zu Berlin, Breslau und Wilna gemachte rhinoplastische Operationen, *J. Chir, Augenheilk.* **12,** 630 (1828).

Hospital in London, used platinum in an attempt to prevent the contraction of a reconstructed nose:

Case report The patient was a man aged 27, of scrofulous diathesis, by trade a working goldsmith. His habits had been irregular, but he had not been addicted to intemperance. In 1831 he had gonorrhoea and chancres, for which he took mercury, and apparently got well. But a few weeks later inflammation destroyed part of his soft palate; this was arrested by mercurial fumigations. One year later his nose became swollen and tender, with discharge of pieces of bone. He was treated with mercury and sarsaparilla, but the disease progressed, and he was admitted to St. Thomas's Hospital. His whole nose with the turbinates was lost. Tyrrell prescribed *solut. potassae hydriodatis* (Lugol's); this brought rapid improvement. One year after he was completely healed, the restoration was carried out. A cast, in plaster of Paris, was made of his face, and on this a light but firm frame of platina was formed to support the new nose, but contrived so that it could be easily removed. Tyrrell then modelled wax over this, which, when it had been spread out, was laid on the forehead, and the outline marked in indigo. A flap of this shape was dissected up, leaving little or nothing but the pericranium. Bleeding was controlled with German tinder, which was also used to dress the forehead.[23] The patient bore the operation without a murmur or complaint, and was conveyed to his bed in high spirits. Everything went well for 2–3 weeks, and then the flap started to contract irregularly. Soon the frame projected out of the left nostril, and was easily removed by the patient. After small secondary corrections of lip and alae the nose did not alter. The patient was freed of a hideous deformity and dryness of the pharynx, and his voice was improved.[24]

MAKING THE BRIDGE OF THE NOSE

When from syphilis, or other cause, only the bridge of the nose is missing, and the side-walls and tip are undamaged, it can be reconstructed by a longitudinal strip from the forehead. Dieffenbach described two cases in which the flap was inserted into an incision down the midline of the nose.[25] More recently he has treated a Russian doctor with scrofulous caries, for which he had had three years of

[23] [See p. 174, n. 2.]

[24] [F. Tyrrell, A case of loss of nose, and restoration by the Taliacotian operation, *Lond. med. surg. J.* **6,** 730 (1835).]

[25] Dieffenbach, *Erfahrungen,* Vol. 2, pp. 33–4 (1830).

mercurials. The nasal bones had been destroyed, and the soft tissues had collapsed, forming a deep groove. For nine years this poor fellow had put up with his deformity in solitude. Dieffenbach split the nose, after separating the columella from the tip, and inserted a large oval flap. Later he excised narrow strips from the sides of the flap, until it was the width of a normal bridge. He regarded this as one of his most successful rhinoplasties, for the nose showed hardly a sign of artefact. Von Ammon[26] and others have also used this technique. These cases are similar to the very common saddle-nose, where the cartilaginous support has collapsed (but the skin is normal), which is treated by insetting a flap;[27] the only difference is that this flap is smaller than for the whole nasal bridge.

EXCISION OF TISSUE FOR THE TREATMENT OF SMALL DEPRESSIONS

Dieffenbach was the first to treat small depressions in the cartilaginous part of the nose by excision of tissue, according to the particular case, when the bony bridge is intact.[28]

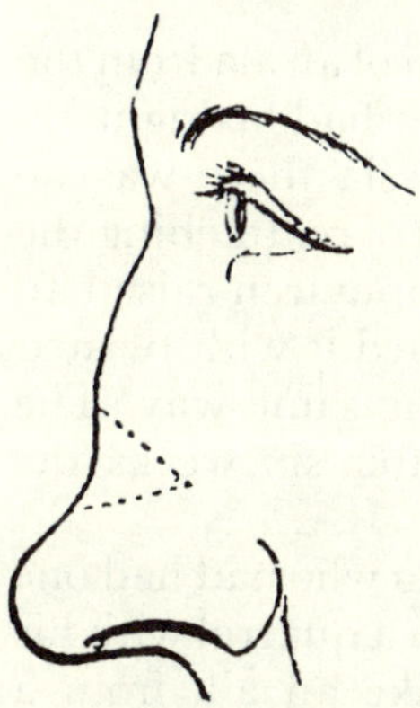

Fig. 19

If the nose is too long for the face, a transverse wedge is removed in full thickness [Fig. 19]. The upper incision, just below the nasal bones, is made first, otherwise it is difficult to steady the tissues for the second incision. A piece of the septum is included, so that it will not project too far. When the bleeding (which is brisk) has stopped, two interrupted sutures are inserted in the septum, and tied; one end is cut short, and the other is brought out through the nostril. The skin is closed with 6–8 twisted sutures.

For smaller noses, an oval is excised in full thickness on both sides; the septum and the skin are sutured as above [Fig. 20]. The lengthening caused by the suture of two curved incisions produces a little lump in the midline, but this later contracts to leave the bridge level. Dieffenbach treated a doctor of philosophy in this way, who had a depressed nose following scrofula in childhood. The width of the piece of tissue excised was one-third of an inch. After four weeks the bridge was level, and there were only fine scars to be seen. The patient was delighted.[29]

---

[26] Von Ammon, Morioplastik, p. 162 (1830).

[27] See p. 92.

[28] Dieffenbach, *Erfahrungen*, Vol. 2, p. 1 (1830).

[29] Ibid, p. 9.

If the nose is so small that no tissue can be removed from the bridge, smaller ovals are excised [Fig. 21]. A woman aged 44 had been cured of a syphilitic ulcer of the nose by careful treatment with mercury. After the ovals had been excised, it was possible to see right through the nose. Two sutures that were left until the fifth day cut out, and a small hole was left on one side; this was healed in two weeks with silver nitrate. The bridge of the nose was completely restored.[30]

RECONSTRUCTION OF THE ALA

Dieffenbach was the first to reconstruct individual parts of the nose, but his attempts to build an ala from the cheek were not very successful, as the nostril contracted. The skin of the cheek is unsuitable for transplantation because of this tendency to contract. Dieffenbach then took the skin from the forehead; although the pedicle must be quite long, and the side-wall of the nose has to be split in its full length, he prefers it to the cheek.[31] He sometimes uses the cheek for small defects of the posterior part of the ala, following caries of the maxilla.

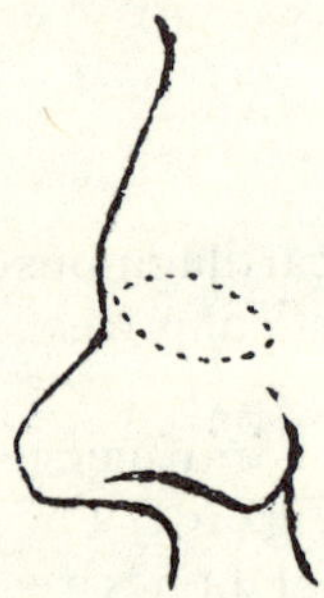

Fig. 20

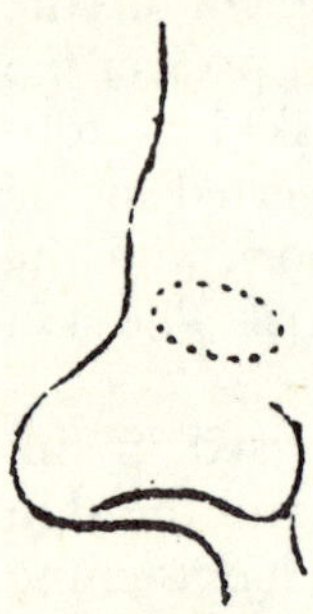

Fig. 21

Labat described the reconstruction of an ala from the cheek by Dupuytren:[32] a Polish officer had his right ala slashed off. On the retreat to Prussia there was no medical attention, and no possibility of reattaching the fragment. On 23 November 1832 Dupuytren raised an oval flap from the cheek, and attached it with twisted sutures. The cheek was closed in the same way. The pedicle smoothed itself out, and after six weeks the repair could hardly be seen.

Jobert also used the cheek for a man who had had one ala and the tip of his nose bitten off in a quarrel with his beloved.[33] Dzondi's attempt to make an ala from a completely detached piece of skin from another person was a failure.[34] The problem of the contracture of the skin of the cheek (because of its thinness) can be overcome by doubling it over. The flap must be made correspondingly larger than the defect, and the edge is then turned in and sutured before the flap is inset.

[30] Ibid, p. 10.

[31] Ibid. pp. 27–9.

[32] Labat, *De la rhinoplastie*, p. 245.

[33] Jobert [case demonstration], *Gaz, Méd.* p. 76 (1836).

[34] See p. 84.

RECONSTRUCTION OF THE SIDE-WALL OF THE NOSE

Loss of one ala is often combined with loss of the side-wall of the nose. Reconstruction is required, not only for appearance, but to prevent involvement of the lacrimal apparatus, and for fear that exposure of the nasal bone will lead to its exfoliation. Delpech has successfully replaced one wall of the nose and part of the lower eyelid with a forehead flap.[35] He did this and other plastic operations as early as 1820, and it is a wonder that this did not inspire his countrymen, for only now are they showing more enthusiasm for this branch of surgery. The part of the flap over the nasal bone will adhere by its under-surface as well as by its margins. But the lower part, forming the ala, has a free inner surface, and it is much more difficult to prevent contraction of the new nostril margin. Although I have no personal experience of the technique, I would recommend that the edge of the flap should be doubled over. The other details of the operative technique are unnecessary for anyone who knows how to do a rhinoplasty, and who understands the general rules for transplantation. Defects differ so much that the method must be altered to suit each case. Plastic operations give the surgeon much more scope for ingenuity than other operations where the anatomical considerations are all the same, e.g. amputations, ligature of vessels, etc.

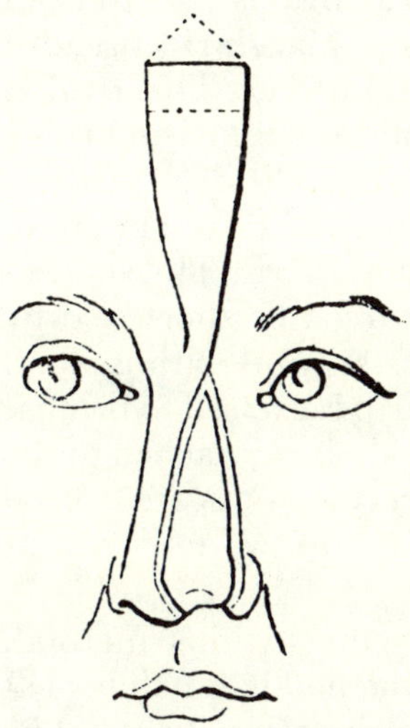

Fig. 22

Figure 22 is an imaginary drawing of the design of a forehead flap to replace the side of the nose (similar to Delpech's case). If I had a defect like this to treat, I would make a paper pattern of the flap, which in its lower part is the same size as the upper part of the nose, but in its upper part (which will make the ala) is larger in all dimensions, so that the nostril will not be too small, and its margin can be doubled over. The defect should always be prepared first, so that it will not be obscured by blood from the forehead, and so that its exact size can be measured. This is often much larger than it appears at first, even when quite narrow strips are excised, and it may be necessary to alter the pattern. The suturing starts by turning in the free border (indicated by the dotted line), and sewing its raw surfaces together as one would stitch a mattress.

[35] Delpech, *Chirurgie clinique,* Vol. 2, p. 221.

SMALL DEFECTS IN THE NOSTRIL MARGINS

Even small defects in the nostril margin constitute a deformity by giving the patient a somewhat sinister appearance; large defects are as horrible as any other major loss of tissue. If the defect is not more than a quarter of an inch in a smallish nose, Dieffenbach's practice is to reduce the opposite ala and the septum, and to lengthen the defective side, by incising the dorsum of the nose, completely splitting the cartilaginous part. The incision is continued through the tip, separating the defective ala from it, and the tissues are divided from the nasal bone, so that the whole side of the nose can be pulled down. Then an oval is excised from the middle of the normal side, parallel to the nostril margin; its breadth should be about half the breadth of the original defect. This oval is closed with three or four interrupted sutures, and the split nasal bridge is repaired with a row of twisted sutures. During this, the deformed ala is pulled down until it is a little longer than the normal side. The small prominent tip of the flap must be trimmed with scissors. The septum then projects too far in front of the alae, and it must be shortened by separating the columella from the cartilaginous septum with a small knife. The cartilage is held with forceps, and a strip is excised to bring it into the correct relationship with the alae. The skin is reattached to the cartilage with sutures. All this constitutes a very complicated nasal wound, and strenuous measures must be taken to prevent inflammation.

Dieffenbach has restored a number of patients by this method, including a handsome young Prussian uhlan, who had had half his left ala bitten off by his horse. If the ala is completely missing it should be replaced from the forehead, cheek, or lip. For very narrow defects Dieffenbach excises the margins, as for a hare-lip, and closes the wound with twisted sutures. If this narrows the nostril, he puts in one of my rubber tubes for a time, or enlarges the opening by incising the junction of the nostril with the upper lip. If he has to take a larger wedge out of one ala, he excises a similar piece from the normal side to make them equal. With broader defects this would depress the tip of the nose. He therefore lengthens the defective side, and removes a piece from the bridge and the septum. When this has healed, he excises an equal amount from the normal side. He has treated several people by this method, either after excision of cancer or after accidental wounding, and they have been so perfectly healed that there is no scar to be seen.[36]

---

[36] Dieffenbach, *Erfahrungen*, Vol. 5 (1838) [unpublished].

BUILDING UP A COLLAPSED NOSE

When the supporting bone and cartilage have been destroyed, but the skin is mostly intact, the surgeon has to decide whether to excise any remnants that would interfere with a conventional rhinoplasty, or to keep them, and, if necessary, replace only a small part by skin from a distance. Dieffenbach's policy is to keep them.[37] The patient's head is held by an assistant, and an incision with a narrow pointed scalpel in the left nostril divides the soft tissues up to the nasal process of the frontal bone. A similar incision is made on the right side (see Fig. 12). The central strip *a* consists of the bridge and tip of the old nose, attached above to the forehead, and below to the contracted columella and the upper lip. The columella is lengthened by an incision in the lip on each side. The side-walls of the nose are raised as two lateral flaps *bb* with one border where the nose joins the cheek. They are completely freed by semicircular incisions at the attachment of the alae, and then carefully separated from the bone. The skin of the cheek on each side is now undermined so that it can later be advanced medially to prevent the newly raised nose spreading sideways.

The actual build-up of the nose now starts by cutting the edges of the central flap with scissors in such a way that the inner surface is narrower than the outer, and the flap becomes triangular in cross-section, like the keystone of an arch (*a*) [Fig. 23]. Nothing is removed from the epidermal surface. The lateral flaps are treated in the opposite way, by removing a strip from the outer surface, leaving the inner intact (*bb*). On the straight edges straight scissors are used, and on the alar margins ophthalmic scissors curved on the flat. The nasal incisions are closed with twisted sutures. A stitch is put through the part of the upper lip from which the columella has been lifted; when this is tied it brings the lip behind the columella, pushing it and the tip of the nose forwards. The nose is joined to the cheeks with interrupted sutures. Finally, the new base for the nose (*cc*) is established by passing two long needles through the cheeks, under the nose, and twisting their ends up over strips of leather.[38]

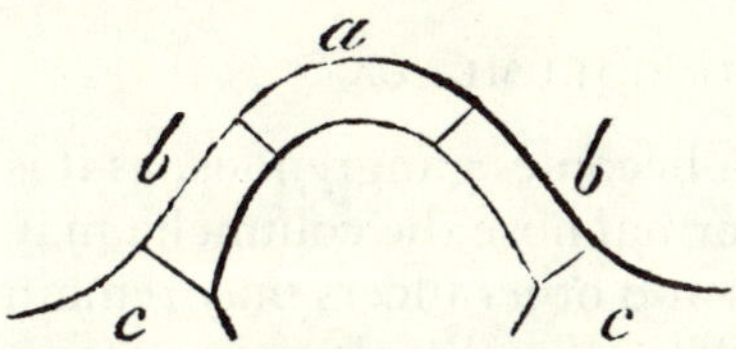

Fig. 23

Nowadays Dieffenbach treats most of these cases by insetting and burying a flap;[39] these noses are more solid and less likely to collapse

37 Dieffenbach, *Erfahrungen*, Vol. 1, p. 9 (1829).

38 [See also p. 91.]

39 [See p. 94.]

again. For the after-treatment he used to recommend fomentations of tepid wine, but he has changed this to a vigorous anti-inflammatory regime.

THE CROOKED NOSE

The depression of the tip of the nose in most patients with double hare-lip and cleft palate, and the obliquity of the nose in simple clefts, are due to a fold in the cartilaginous septum; this prevents free elevation of the tip of the nose, even though it may be somewhat improved by the hare-lip operation. Dividing this fold corrects the deformity: the columella is held aside, the fold is pierced with the tip of a small scalpel, and the cartilage is divided up to its junction with the bony septum. The tip of the nose then comes up on its own, and can be lifted even further. If nothing more is done, the deformity will recur, particularly as elevation is limited by the intact columella. The tip must therefore be held forward by compression of the nose from side to side; this will open up the incision in the cartilage, and the space will be filled with granulations. A lead plate can be bent and worn on the nose like a saddle. Dieffenbach uses small pieces of lead or leather, through which long insect-pins are passed; the ends of these are twisted up, and they can safely be left in place for 2–3 weeks.[40]

RECONSTRUCTION OF THE COLUMELLA

Sometimes in a rhinoplasty the columella becomes gangrenous, as it is the part furthest from the pedicle. In a normal nose the columella may be the only part to be destroyed; herpetic and other ulcers may remain localized there. But in a wound, loss of the columella alone is uncommon, as the rest of the nose is usually damaged at the same time. It would be too much of an undertaking to replace the columella from the forehead when the nose-tip is present—the nose would have to be split in its full length. There is enough local tissue available.

The columella may be reconstructed as part of a rhinoplasty. Apart from improving the appearance of the nose, the columella helps to support the tip. In the Italian and Gräfe's methods the necessary skin is taken from the base of the flap after it has healed soundly to the face, and has been separated from the arm. Gräfe's modification of the Taliacotian operation shortens its stages, and he attaches the columella as soon as it has been fashioned. In the Indian operation it is quite often

[40] Dieffenbach, *Erfahrungen*, Vol. 2, p. 15 (1830).

necessary to use hairy scalp to get enough length for the columella, which should be one inch broad. The growth of hair gradually stops with repeated plucking, and the thick skin of the scalp is ideal. Most surgeons attach the columella at the same time as the rest of the flap; only Lisfranc leaves it until later, putting lead tubes in the nose until then. The columella is raised with a triangular extension, which is then cut off transversely. This makes it easier to close the defect in the forehead, but Dieffenbach thinks that it is wasteful to throw away this little piece of skin. If part of the old columella remains, the new one can be that much smaller. If it is completely missing, and there is a shortage of skin on the forehead, it can be reconstructed separately, before the main operation, from a piece of the old nose that is not being used, or from the upper lip; if this is successful, the forehead flap can be smaller.

Case report Von Ammon had a patient for rhinoplasty, whose upper lip was split in the middle like a hare-lip. As the forehead was very low he took a half-inch strip of the full thickness of one side of the cleft, rotated it up so that its epidermal surface was still on the outside, and then repaired the lip. The rotation must have put too much strain on the pedicle, for the flap became gangrenous. There was nothing for it but to make the columella out of the scalp, in the course of the rhinoplasty. But this also necrosed, and von Ammon later took another flap from the upper lip. This time he turned it directly upwards, so that the mucosal surface was on the outside. At first it healed well, and looked just like a normal columella, but after a year it had separated from the lip, and was nourished entirely by the tip of the nose. However, the gap was hardly noticeable, and it was not necessary to reattach it.

Reconstruction from the nose

If the nose is very large, so that the removal of a piece might actually improve it, and the upper lip is scarred or short, reconstruction from the nose is indicated. Dieffenbach's technique is to take a flap one inch long and one-third of an inch wide (based on the nose-tip), which he rotates, and sets into the upper lip. The flap is pointed, and its terminal triangle is excised [Fig. 24]. The nose is repaired with twisted sutures. The little lump that remains on the tip of the nose can be excised later.[41]

Another method, also by Dieffenbach, is to raise a flap on the lower part of the nose, and to move it down without rotation. This is most

[41] C. Tax, *De septi narium restitutione,* Diss., Berlin, (1836).

suitable for a drooping or a saddle-shaped nose [Fig. 25]. The incisions are carried down to the free border of the nasal opening. The lower part of the flap is pared in preparation, and the flap is freed, leaving only its inferior attachment to nourish it. It is now usually mobile enough to be

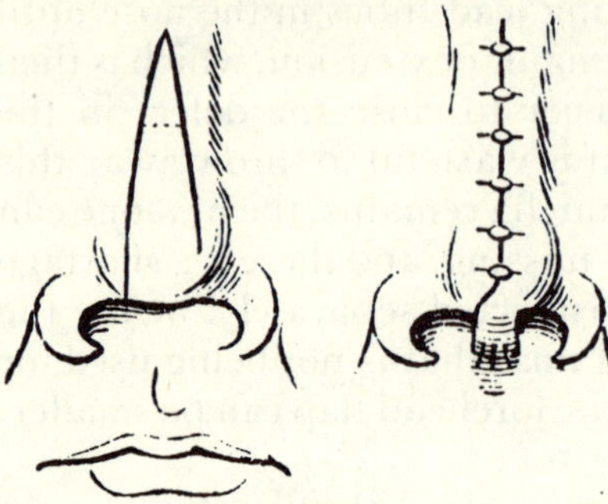

Fig. 24

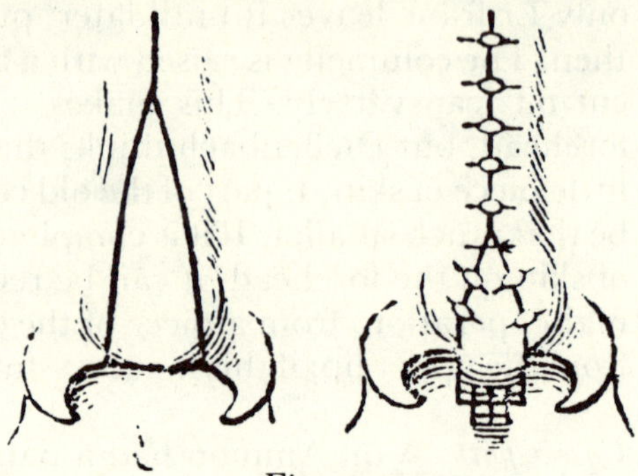

Fig. 25

brought down to the upper lip; if not, the cartilage of the tip of the nose and the septum must be incised transversely until the lower part of the flap meets the incision in the upper lip. The columella is attached to the lip with interrupted sutures, and the nose is repaired with twisted sutures which include the pointed tip of the flap forming the upper part of the columella. This prevents the flap returning to its old site.[42] But it is as well to cover the whole nose-tip with plaster, fixed to the cheeks near the upper lip, so that the new columella is not stretched by the elasticity of the nasal cartilage.

Reconstruction from the upper lip

If the nose is small or deformed, the columella can be reconstructed by taking a flap in full thickness from the upper lip, and repairing the lip as for a hare-lip. The red margin is excised, and the flap is either rotated up to the nose-tip, or turned straight up so that the mucosa is on the outside. The latter is preferable, as the texture of the mucosa soon changes and it comes to look like skin, and the flap does not have to be turned through two right-angles. This is supported by Fricke,[43] and by Dieffenbach, especially for men with thick upper lips. Dieffenbach has also produced very good-looking columellas from dense scarring of the

[42] [See p. 96, n. 28.]

[43] J. C. G. Fricke, Wiederersatz des knorpeligen Theils eines gänzlich zerstörten Septum narium aus der Oberlippe, *J. Chir. Augenheilk.* **22,** 456 (1834).

upper lip, which would have justified excision as for cancer. In one patient, after a successful reconstruction from a scar of the lip, he had to excise a carcinoma of the columella.[44]

If the upper lip is very broad, and the skin of the nose-tip is thin, with collapsed alae, the nose can be given greater stability by Dieffenbach's technique: after the flap has been raised from the full thickness of the lip, the red margin is not excised, but an incision is made in the skin just above the skin–vermilion junction, through the skin and subcutaneous tissue, without damaging the mucosa. If the flap is now turned straight up, there is a little flap attached to it by mucosa, with a raw surface that can be sutured to the under-surface of the nose-tip.

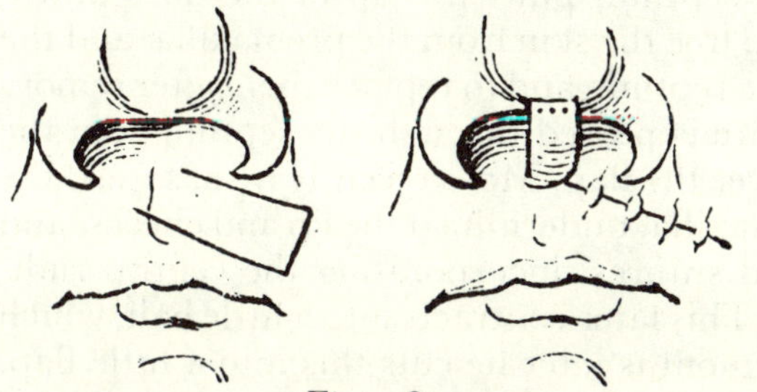

Fig. 26

Another method is to make a flap of the skin only. The lip must be long enough to withstand such a defect. The pattern is placed transversely on the lip, and a flap about one and a quarter inches long and half an inch wide is turned through a right angle [Fig. 26]. If the cartilaginous septum is present (as it usually is in these cases), sutures are passed through it, and tied over the new columella to hold the raw surfaces together.

Fergusson, in an account of a rhinoplasty, has mentioned Liston's method of making the columella from the upper lip,[45] but I have no further information on this.[46]

Reconstruction by the Italian method

Labat reported reconstruction of the columella from the thenar eminence of the hand.[47] The small size of the flap required allows this site to

[44] Dieffenbach, *Erfahrungen*, Vol. 5 (1838) [unpublished].

[45] W. Fergusson, Case of reparation of the nose, *Edinb. med. surg. J.* **43,** 363 (1835) [building up the nose by Dieffenbach's method for collapse due to syphilis.]

[46] [Robert Liston (1794–1847), surgeon, Royal Infirmary, Edinburgh (1827), and University College Hospital, London (1834), had described five cases of reconstruction of the columella from the upper lip, in which he turned the flap straight up through 180°. He was probably the first to do this. See his: Operation for restoring the columna nasi, *Edinb. med. surg. J.* **35,** 84 (1831).]

[47] Labat, *De la rhinoplastie*, p. 256. [This seems to have been only a suggestion of Labat's, and he never actually carried it out.]

be used, rather than the upper arm. The position of the arm is also much more comfortable than in the usual Italian method.

LENGTHENING THE COLUMELLA

If the new columella is too short, it can be lengthened by making a quarter of an inch incision in each nostril, meeting in a 'V'. This frees the columella from the lip, but it must not be freed any further from its bed. The tip of the nose can now be lifted and held in this position with sticking-plaster; the little wound will heal by granulation. If the central element is removed in a double hare-lip, the loss of the premaxilla, usually with a piece of the septum, pulls the tip of the nose down. Dieffenbach's technique is to free the skin from the premaxilla, and the shortened columella from the septum, and to replace them after removing the premaxilla.[48] A suture is passed through the septum, and the ends are knotted together over the flap. More recently he has freed the upper lip, removed the premaxilla, undermined the lip and cheeks, and closed the cleft with twisted sutures, incorporating the central rudiment of the lip in the repair. This later contracts into a little ball, which is what he intends. Several months later he cuts this into a little flap, makes a transverse incision immediately under the nose (a 'moustache' incision, as he calls it), and fixes the edge of the flap to the upper lip with two fine sutures. In this way he has so perfectly restored large numbers of grossly deformed children that no trace of their deformity can be seen.[49]

CLOSING HOLES IN THE NOSE

This is not as difficult as closing holes in cavities that contain fluid, for the nasal mucus escapes through the nostrils, and does not interfere with healing. But it is still not as easy as one might hope. When the edges are excised and sutured, the problem is that the skin over the hole has no backing; it sinks into the cavity, so that the edges are not as exactly apposed as they should be. But this only happens with interrupted sutures. Twisted sutures are much surer, holding the skin out of the cavity, and keeping the edges raised in a seam, which then levels out when the pins are removed. Although Rust regards this as a plastic operation,[50] this is not strictly correct, since no new tissue is brought

48 Dieffenbach, *Erfahrungen*, Vol. 2, p. 20 (1830).

49 Ibid. Vol. 5 (1838) [unpublished].

50 See n. 20 above.

into the defect. However, there are some cases where the opening is so large that this is necessary. A small hole may heal naturally, but, if it is larger, the margins will become scarred over before it can fill with granulations.

In other parts of the body, where the tissues are thicker, the process of healing is the same, but the healing comes not only from the margins but also from granulations sprouting from the whole floor of the wound. Sometimes a broad or a depressed scar remains, but it never leaves a hole. The size and shape of the defect in the nose will determine whether the skin is taken from the nose, the face, or the forehead. Dieffenbach has done many of these operations, and has then later smoothed out a flap that has contracted into a ball, or excised it completely to bring the original margins together. In this way he has successfully closed a large hole into the frontal sinus. Syme has recently published a similar operation.[51]

SECONDARY CORRECTION OF RECONSTRUCTED NOSES

Tagliacozzi described the need for secondary correction, using external splints and internal tubes, continued for several years.[52] I have already discussed how the effect of these disappears soon after they are removed.[53] He also recommended that pale or discoloured noses should be tanned in the midday or afternoon sun. The face should not be exposed for more than ½–1 hour, or it would harm the head, but this could be repeated frequently. To improve the texture of reconstructed parts, and to soften scars, he advised ox- or calf bile, and particularly the bile of a tortoise. The fat of a donkey and many other things, especially preparations of lead, were famous for narrowing broad scars. Depressed scars with raised margins were levelled by binding on lead plates. If the scar was too hard to respond to this, it was scarified so that the groove became filled with granulations. If that was not enough, the whole scar was excised and re-sutured, with the warning that the new scar might be raised instead of depressed. This all shows that the old Master of plastic surgery was an expert at the secondary correction of his new noses. He put his faith in many remedies that no one wishes to try nowadays, but, when they failed, he too had recourse to the knife.

It is perfectly true that Dieffenbach's principle of making the flap too large, and removing the excess later, creates the need for secondary

---

[51] See p. 52, n. 13.

[52] Tagliacozzi, *de curtorum,* Vol. 2, Chapter 17.

[53] See p. 42.

operations. But this does not invalidate the principle. When the flap is too small it certainly saves another operation, but there is then nothing that can be done to improve it. What Labat says is not true: 'one can very rarely persuade the patient to be cut again.'[54] I have never yet seen a patient, having gone through the pain of a rhinoplasty, who has then refused the minor improvements needed for his new nose, even if these have to be carried out with the knife. These small secondary operations are mainly excisions of unsightly scars and removal of excess tissue. Nature is very active in narrowing scars, and there is often no need to excise a scar that started by being broad, for it will contract, and become paler, and later may be hardly noticeable.

But there are many occasions when healing has been by granulation and not by first intention. If florid granulations are not destroyed by cauterization, there will be a raised scar. This can be excised by two parallel incisions through the full thickness of the skin, meeting exactly at a point at each end; the wound is closed with twisted sutures. A depressed scar is more difficult to deal with; it commonly occurs after the edge of a flap has become gangrenous, or has healed after suppuration, but with poor granulations. Simple excision does not help, for the surrounding skin is adherent to the underlying tissues. These adhesions must be divided by undermining the edges of the wound on both sides. If necessary, the scar can be excised with the knife directed obliquely, so that more of the deeper tissue is removed, and more of the epidermal surface is retained. This provides an excess of skin, which helps to overcome the depression. Dieffenbach treats small irregularities in the skin by scarification. He also scarifies both sides of the nose to make the tip more prominent; the raw surfaces are treated with cold water and then with lead lotion.

Removal of excess tissue includes excision of the rotated pedicle, and of other parts of the flap that are too large. This can only be done by excising skin vertically in full thickness, and then carefully suturing the wound; horizontal excision leaves a broad ugly scar. The scalpel is inserted at right angles through the skin, the handle is lowered, and two curved incisions are made, which meet exactly at the ends without crossing. Experience will soon show what shape to make this—a narrow ellipse, like a myrtle leaf, or broader, more oval, or even circular. If there is any doubt, a narrow strip should be taken first, and the wound edges approximated; more skin can then be removed if necessary.

One important rule is that the excision must always run in the long axis of the nose. This produces a slight lengthening of the nose, and

---

[54] See p. 87.

pushes the tip forwards, whereas transverse incisions have the opposite effect. When two curved incisions are brought together to make a straight line, the wound will be longer than before. Even if it contracts later, and to some extent evens this out, the advantage of a longitudinal scar is obvious.

Other secondary operations include making the nose-tip more prominent,[55] and restoring and lengthening the columella. The after-care is the same as for all plastic operations, but the wounds from these secondary procedures are so small that they do not cause any general reaction. The wound must not be sutured until all bleeding has stopped and the serous stage is reached; it will then usually heal by first intention.

In many cases Dieffenbach excises the scar left on the forehead after a rhinoplasty. The original wound can easily be sutured at its upper and lower ends, but there is a gap of 2–3 inches in the middle; this can be made smaller by advancing the skin, but the rest must be left to heal by granulation. Repeated applications of silver nitrate to the exuberant granulations will encourage contraction, but a large flap still leaves a considerable scar. Sometimes this takes on the colour of the surrounding skin, but it may remain dark red or blueish, with little vessels in it, so that it is visible from a distance. If the patient is willing, or if he can be persuaded by the surgeon, there is no danger in excising this scar. An incision is made round it, and it is freed from the frontal bone; it is more densely adherent than the normal skin of the forehead, which is separated from the bone by connective tissue. The skin is pulled together, and undermined a little if necessary, or, if the tension is still too great, lateral relieving incisions are made. Closure by twisted sutures results in a very neat scar. This answers the criticism of the Indian operation (as compared with the Italian), that it leaves a disfiguring scar on the forehead.

[55] See p. 96, n. 28.

12

EYELID—BLEPHAROPLASTY

Blepharoplasty is the part of plastic surgery concerned with the reconstruction of eyelids that have been completely destroyed. In the earlier surgical writings, which include reconstruction of the nose and the lip, there is no mention of the eyelid, and it is only with the resurgence of plastic surgery in this [nineteenth] century that eyelids, as well as other parts of the body, have been restored. The term 'blepharoplasty' has become so popular recently that it has been applied not only to reconstruction but to other smaller operations on the lids, such as the correction of ectropion. Jäger's operation, as described in Dreyer's dissertation,[1] is not a true blepharoplasty but a method of treating lagophthalmos.[2] But even if it is restricted to operations where a piece of skin is transplanted, a distinction must be made between complete loss of the lid and partial loss, where tissue remains that can be used for reconstruction. This distinction is more important in blepharoplasty than in rhinoplasty. In rhinoplasty, the question of removal of remnants of the old nose may be determined by the general principle that no part of the human body should be removed unnecessarily. In blepharoplasty, however, it is a positive advantage to retain any parts of the old lid, so that it need not be completely reconstructed. For this is a very difficult task. The eyelids are made up of many different tissues, with glands, cartilage, lashes, and special musculature, and they are responsible for the protection of the eye. They are closely connected with the lacrimal apparatus, and this and the eye will be affected if the lids are not functioning. It is impossible to re-create such a complicated structure, as skin is the only tissue available for the reconstruction. The result must be imperfect, and it is enough if vision is improved and the eye is protected from too much light and air. This is all that can be expected of plastic surgery at the present time; the functions of the lashes, glands, and tear-duct must remain unrestored. It is the same with the muscles, so that reconstruction of the upper lid is much more difficult than the lower, which is less mobile. A new upper lid is often

[1] J. T. Dreyer, *Nova blepharoplastices methodus*, Diss., Vienna (1831).

[2] [Inability to close the eye, but without eversion of the lid.]

either too short, so that the eye cannot be closed, or too long and immobile, so that it hangs down, and interferes with vision.

EARLY ATTEMPTS

Gräfe was the first to state that the technique of nasal reconstruction could be applied to the eyelid. He described the case of a Jewish girl with destruction of the eyelid by gangrene following erysipelas. But all he says of the operation is that he turned up a piece of the skin of the adjoining cheek, with a very satisfactory result.[3]

Dzondi treated eyelids contracted by scar-tissue, by simply dividing the scar and allowing it to heal by granulation.[4] But anyone who has tried this will know that, even if it produces a broader scar at first, the contracture gradually recurs. This is not really plastic surgery. But another of his operations, in 1818, deserves the title of blepharoplasty:

Case report An officer had lost the greater part of one lower eyelid from infection following a wound. Dzondi first excised the overgrown conjunctiva at the inner canthus. To reconstruct the lid he made a curved incision in the cheek outwards from the inner canthus, half an inch below and parallel to the defect. An incision was made at right angles to the outer end of this, and a flap one and a half inches long and half an inch wide was lifted and sutured to the remnant of the lid at the outer canthus. The defect in the cheek was left to granulate. Healing was incomplete, and small secondary operations were needed. The new lid was still not high enough, although it retained the tears. Dzondi therefore used his earlier technique to raise it; this took four weeks to heal. The lid also did not lie close enough to the globe; this was not due to the laxity of the flap, but to swelling of the conjunctiva. This was controlled by cauterization, with careful protection of the eye. Finally Dzondi tried to implant eyelashes, but without success. The new lid matched the other, controlled the flow of tears, and protected the eye.[5]

It can be seen that this technique is only suitable for cases where part of the old lid remains; it is still very different from the true blepharoplasty—the construction of a whole new lid.

---

[3] Gräfe, *Rhinoplastik*, p. 15. [The patient was treated in 1809.]

[4] C. H. Dzondi, *Beiträgen zur Vervollkommnung der Heilkunde*, Vol. 1, Halle, p. 166 (1816).

[5] C. H. Dzondi, Bildung eines neuen unteren Augenlides aus der Wange, *J. prakt. Heilk.* **47**, 99 (1818).

Fricke's method[6]

This is really meant for severe ectropion. Excess conjunctiva is first reduced by medicaments or by excision. When this has healed, the scar holding the lid is excised, or, if it is narrow and not too hard, it is divided by an incision parallel to the lid margin, and as far away from it as possible. The most difficult cases are those where the lid is adherent to the orbital margin. Here the incision is started in the centre, and extended laterally and then medially. The wound edges are held apart by assistants, and the subcutaneous tissues and the orbicularis are divided up to the conjunctiva, which is carefully preserved. It is a great advantage for the future mobility of the lid if the orbicularis can be saved, but the incision must go deep enough to make room for the flap.

For the upper lid the flap is taken from the forehead, and for the lower lid from the cheek. If the flap is too close to the orbital margin the contraction of the scar will reproduce the ectropion.

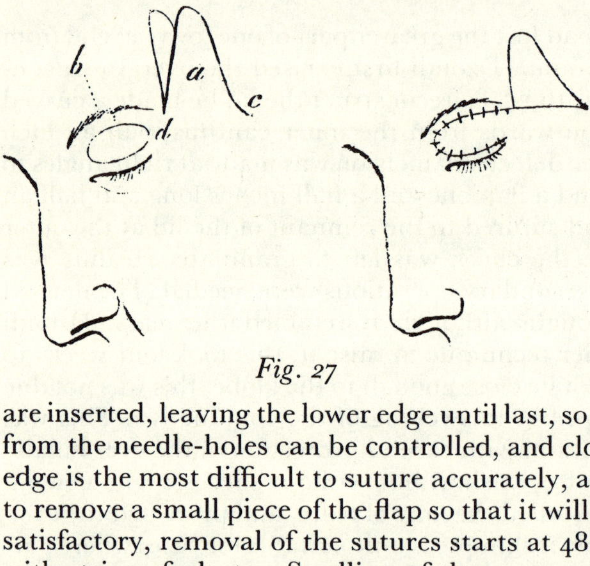

Fig. 27

The size of the flap (*a*) is measured and marked out [Fig. 27]. The incision (*c*) is curved outwards, and the bridge of skin (*d*) is excised, to allow the flap to rotate into the defect (*b*) without tension. After the bleeding has been controlled, interrupted sutures are inserted, leaving the lower edge until last, so that any fresh bleeding from the needle-holes can be controlled, and clots removed. The inner edge is the most difficult to suture accurately, and it may be necessary to remove a small piece of the flap so that it will lie evenly. If healing is satisfactory, removal of the sutures starts at 48 hours, replacing them with strips of plaster. Swelling of the new eyelid is treated with *Aq. Goulardi*,[7] and small unhealed suppurating areas are dressed with *unguentum nigrum*.[8]

---

[6] J. C. G. Fricke, *Die Bildung neuer Augenlider (Blepharoplastik) nach Zerstörungen*, Hamburg (1829).

[7] [Lead sub-acetate.]

[8] [Zinc ointment, balsam of Peru, and powdered silver nitrate.]

Case report Fricke used this method in 1829 for a man with severe ectropion of the left upper lid following a burn. The lid was so distorted that the tips of the lashes touched his eyebrow. Exposure of the globe was causing opacity of the cornea. At operation the scarred muscle was divided down to the conjunctiva. Because of scarring on the temple, a flap was raised on the cheek, with a relatively wide pedicle. The next day the whole area was red and very swollen, and this did not settle for six days. The tip of the flap became gangrenous, and separated. The swollen conjunctiva was treated with *tinct. opii*, and, later, part of it was excised, and the wound healed with *aqua Conradi*.[9] The patient was much improved, for the new eyelid perfectly fulfilled its function, and the corneal opacity, the redness, and the swelling of the conjunctiva disappeared.

Jüngken recommended a similar technique for lagophthalmos, as all the methods up to that time had given such poor results. The only difference was that his flap had a narrower pedicle than Fricke's. His recommendation was made before he knew of Fricke's work, and he operated on two patients: a scrofulous boy with his lower eyelid so distorted by gangrenous erysipelas that the tarsal margin was adherent to the orbital margin, and a second boy in the same condition after a scorpion bite. Both operations were a complete failure.[10]

DIEFFENBACH'S METHOD OF BLEPHAROPLASTY

The only true blepharoplasty is Dieffenbach's method of transposing a flap.[11] Von Ammon has confirmed the excellence of this method from his own experience.[12] Chelius, Eckström, Lisfranc, and other surgeons have also carried it out successfully. It is indicated when the eyelid is either completely missing or cannot be used in the repair, and where the lid margin, which is essential for Fricke's technique, cannot be preserved.

For reconstruction of either lid, Dieffenbach starts by preserving as much of the conjunctiva as possible (if it is not too diseased), and undermining it up to the orbital margin. But if, as often happens, it is

[9] [Corrosive sublimate and *tinct. opii* in distilled water.]

[10] J. C. Jüngken, *Die Lehre von den Augenoperationen*, Berlin, pp. ix, 267 (1829).

[11] J. F, Dieffenbach, Einige Bemerkungen aus und über Paris. Ueber einen Fall von Blepharoplastik, *Caspers Wschr.*, p. 8 (1835) [the first account of the technique of transposition].

[12] F. A. von Ammon, Dr. Dieffenbach's neue Methode der Blepharoplastik, Ein Sendschreiben an Dr. Fricke, *Z. Ophthal.* **4**, 428 (1835).

involved in the malignant process, it is removed with the rest of the lid. Reconstruction is still possible, but it is a great advantage if the conjunctiva can be retained to line the new lid.

The whole diseased lid is now removed by straight incisions from the inner and outer angles of the eye, meeting at a point on the cheek for the lower lid, and on the forehead over the eyebrow for the upper, and including healthy skin at the apex of the triangle [Fig. 28]. The nerves in this region must be preserved as far as possible. For either lid, a horizontal incision is made from the outer canthus over the zygomatic process in the direction of the external auditory meatus; this must be at least one and a half inches long, and, in any case, longer than the width of the defect. From the outer end of this, an incision (into the cheek for the lower lid, and into the temple for the upper) is made parallel to the side of the defect, extending to the level of the tip of the triangle; this incision may get closer to the tip, but not further away. The flap is raised with light strokes of the knife. When the bleeding has been controlled, clots are removed, and the flap is moved sideways into the defect. Since there is no actual rotation, this flap can have a much broader pedicle than one that has to be turned through 90–180°. The corner of the flap, *a*, is fixed into the inner canthus with one interrupted suture. If the conjunctiva has been retained, it is now fixed to the new lid with evenly spaced interrupted sutures; twisted sutures are used for the medial border of the flap. The upper outer corner is held to the outer canthus with one suture, so that the flap does not pull away. The secondary defect on the cheek or the temple will heal by granulation; it is covered with lint, and left to suppurate. It will contract, and the neighbouring skin, particularly the new eyelid, will be pulled on, so that only a very small triangle of scar will be left. In one case in the Charité, however, a whole reconstructed upper lid was destroyed by hospital gangrene.

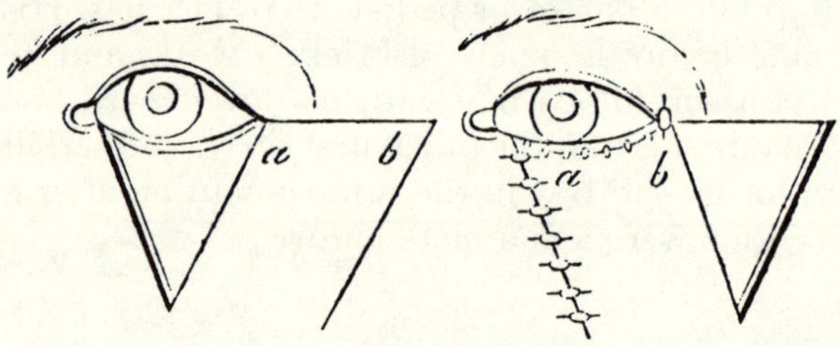

Fig. 28

In recent years Dieffenbach has treated a number of patients by this method, and some of them now look completely normal. In one case he reconstructed both eyelids, with an amazing result. The technique can be used for half a lid, or half the upper and half the lower lid at the same time. He always retains as much of the old lid as possible—small pieces of the tarsal margin with lashes (which will improve the final appearance), and especially the whole tarsal margin, even if it is contracted or adherent to the bone.

For severe ectropion of both lids at the outer canthus, he excises the everted canthus, with a piece of the healthy skin of the temple, as a triangle with its apex towards the ear. Then he makes a curved incision over the supraorbital ridge, and another, one and a half inches below the globe, as far as the nose. The two half-moon shaped tongues are completely undermined, and, by suturing the wound in the temple, they are brought up into place as eyelids, and the conjunctiva is turned inwards.

The earlier methods of blepharoplasty, compared to the true blepharoplasty, are like insetting a flap in the nose compared to full rhinoplasty. They assume that part of the old eyelid remains and can be used in the repair, particularly the conjunctiva and the lid margin. One major disadvantage of Fricke's and Jüngken's method is the tendency for the flaps to contract. This is the process that gives prominence to a nose made of skin, but it is a disaster for a part that should remain flat. There is nothing to stop these flaps contracting, for the surrounding tissues are so lax that they can put up no resistance. Even if the result immediately after the operation seems a great success, the flap gradually contracts, and finally comes to sit on the old lid like a pigeon's egg, making the original deformity worse. Dieffenbach's method is free of all these faults. It can be used when the whole lid is missing. Contracture cannot occur because the contracting scar on the temple or cheek keeps the flap stretched out, with its margin close to the globe. The only criticisms that might be made are the limited movement, and the lack of eyelashes and glands, although one would never imagine that these could be restored.

This seems to be the most perfect technique for reconstruction of the eyelid that plastic surgery will ever be able to achieve. The first time that Dieffenbach did this operation he had to improvise the method on a patient whose lower lid had been destroyed by cancer, who was presented to him at Lisfranc's clinic in Paris.[13]

Case reports On 23 February 1835 I watched von Ammon operating on a woman aged 40 with a cancerous ulcer of the right outer canthus, which had been present for six years. Only a third of the lower lid and two-thirds of the upper were unaffected, After the tumour had been excised her appearance was terrifying, for the remaining parts of the

[13] [See n. 11 above.]

lids had retracted, and the eye was completely exposed. Arterial bleeding was controlled by cold water. Reconstruction was by Dieffenbach's method, with a flap from the cheek for the lower lid. This was quickly but carefully undermined, and no vessels needed tying. The remains of the conjunctiva were advanced and sutured to the edge of the flap; this caused the patient severe pain. For the repair of the upper lid it was possible to advance the skin of the lid over the remains of the tarsal plate, and attach the conjunctiva to it, so that no transplantation was needed. Finally the outer canthus was reconstituted by suturing the outer ends of the lids together. All sutures were removed by the fourth day. There was no contraction of the flap, and the defect on the cheek developed good granulations. On 6 March von Ammon carried out two small secondary operations. The result of all this, so painful for the patient, and so arduous (but so rapidly completed) for the surgeon, was very satisfactory. There has been no recurrence, and her appearance is so nearly normal that only a discerning eye can tell what has been done.

In a second case von Ammon used the same method for a woman whose left upper eyelid was adherent to the supraorbital margin as a result of caries of the bone; the cornea was already covered with pannus. The conjunctiva was so diseased that it could not be preserved, and the operation was not a great success. The raw surface of the flap became covered with a membrane similar to mucous membrane, but this tended to adhere to the globe as in symblepharon. This experience led von Ammon to advise that the margin of the lid should always be preserved if possible, for attachment to a flap from the cheek or the temple, as Peters has shown.[14]

Apart from Dieffenbach, Eckström[15] has also reconstructed an upper eyelid, and Fricke[16] and Blasius (two cases)[17] the lower lid. But these all demonstrate that it is much more difficult to reconstruct an upper eyelid than a nose or any other part.

OTHER RECONSTRUCTIVE OPERATIONS

Blandin[18] published a case that he would have done better to keep quiet about: a girl with complete eversion of the lower lid, which he split and repaired with a flap from the temple, two and a half inches long by half

[14] E. O. Peters, *De blepharoplastice*, Diss., Leipzig, p. 42 (1836).

[15] J. Staub, *De blepharoplastice*, Diss, Berlin, p. 100, (1835).

[16] Peters op. cit.

[17] Staub op. cit.

[18] Blandin, *Autoplastie*, p. 5.

an inch wide; this was not sutured but simply held with sticking-plaster. The flap healed perfectly. It is not clear why he did not use Dieffenbach's method, which he should have known about, for Dieffenbach had already demonstrated it in Paris. Boinet[19] has also used Blandin's method. Jobert[20] excised a cancer of the right lower lid; the bulbar conjunctiva was involved, and was separated with difficulty. He raised a triangular flap on the cheek, one and half inches by half an inch, with its base towards the nose and its apex over the zygoma. This was rotated so that its tip reached the external commissure, and held with two twisted sutures. It healed well, and the pedicle was divided three weeks later.

Carron du Villards operated on a young woman with ectropion of the outer angle of the eye following careless treatment of a malignant pustule with caustic potash. His technique seems to have been similar to Dieffenbach's, although the skin was taken from the eyelid itself, rather than from the temple. In a second case the eye had been injured by a piece of glass in childhood. The eye had collapsed, and the lower lid was everted at the inner canthus. Carron freed an adhesion that was preventing movement of the remnant of the eye, and excised a scar of the lid, with great care not to damage the lacrimal sac. Dieffenbach's twisted sutures and Gräfe's ligature-rods were used to close the wounds. The patient's appearance was improved, and she could wear an artificial eye.[21]

ECTROPION AND LAGOPHTHALMOS

Operations for ectropion and lagophthalmos, which consist simply of incising the skin or excising part of the conjunctiva, will not be included here, as they are dealt with in textbooks of ophthalmology. Only those operations will be described that have some relation to plastic surgery.

Dieffenbach's method

The failure of these earlier methods, particularly Adams' V-shaped excision,[22] which sometimes leaves the patient with a coloboma, and

---

[19] A.-A. Boinet, Ectropion considérable suite de brûlure, blépharoplastie, procédé de M. Blandin, guérison', *Gaz, Méd.*, p. 764 (1836).

[20] A.-J. Jobert, Cancer de la paupière inférieure droite, extirpation, blépharoplastie, guérison', *Gaz, Méd.*, p. 404 (1835).

[21] C.-J. Carron du Villards, Restauration des paupières, *Gaz. Hôp. Paris*, p. 8 (1836).

[22] [W. Adams, *Practical observations on ectropium or the eversion of the eyelids, with the description of a new operation for the cure of that disease*, London, p. 4, (1812).]

worse off than before, led Dieffenbach to a quite different technique, by which the tarsus and the conjunctiva are turned inwards and held in place through an external incision. This is ideal for the lower eyelid, which is more commonly affected.

A small knife is inserted a little below the orbital margin (at the outer canthus for the right eye, and at the inner for the left), and moved from left to right parallel to the orbital margin [Fig. 29]. The skin is freed from the tarsus, and the knife is pushed in until the point comes out between the conjunctiva and the globe; this wound is extended to the full length of the external incision, until the lid remains attached only at the outer and inner canthi. Now the conjunctiva attached to the tarsus is pulled into the skin incision with a hook. The wound is closed with very fine insect-pins, with the conjunctiva and the tarsus included between the two skin edges, so that there are three edges to be sutured together.[23]

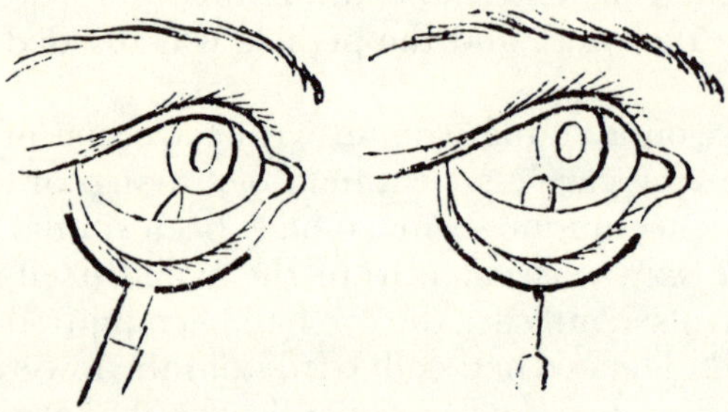

Fig. 29

Ectropion of the upper lid can be treated in the same way. Cold compresses are used to reduce inflammation. There is usually some suppuration, but the operation will be a success if there is adhesion in the depths of the wound.

Case reports Dieffenbach's first patient, treated exactly as above, was a man aged 56 with ectropion of the left lower eyelid from a chronic gonorrhoeal discharge. The operation was followed by severe swelling, which spread out over half the face; this gradually subsided, and the suppurating wound was dressed with *unguentum simplex*,[24] and supported by strips of sticking-plaster. After this, Dieffenbach repeated this operation often, and von Ammon carried it out once. In a woman aged 64, with severe ectropion of the left lower eyelid following a herpetic eruption of the side of her face, Dieffenbach modified his technique by making a V-shaped incision in the skin, extending almost to the middle of the cheek. The vertical part of this was closed with five sutures.[25] This brought about a 'displacement of skin', which supported the eyelid, and prevented it dropping back into its everted

[23] Dieffenbach, *Erfahrungen*, Vol. 2, p. 126 (1830).

[24] [Lard and white wax.]

[25] Dieffenbach, *Erfahrungen*, Vol. 2, p. 131 (1830).

position. This is the same principle as the 'displacement of skin' to lengthen the tip of the nose.[26]

Dieffenbach's more recent methods

Dieffenbach tells me that he has further modified the above operation by making two incisions (*a*, *a*) to raise two flaps on the cheek [Fig. 30]. The edges (*b*, *b*) are joined with twisted sutures, and the edges *ac* and *ca* are joined to the cut margin of the eyelid, pushing this curved incision and the whole lid upwards.

Another of his operations for ectropion is based on the same principle as Dzondi's 'granulation' method,[27] but differs in that the margins of the eyelids are held in the corrected position until healing has taken place. When the deformity is due to contracture of the skin only, this is incised half-way between the free border of the lid and the orbital margin, always following the direction of the fibres of the orbicularis. When the lid has been mobilized in this way, both tarsal margins are freshened, and joined with interrupted sutures, except at the angles, to produce a temporary ankyloblepharon and wide gaping of the incision in the lid. This technique, better than any apparatus, ensures the prolonged closure of the lids. It seems to have no disadvantage for the eye, except that the exclusion of light leads later to transient photophobia. The tears are absorbed normally, and any excess escapes at the inner canthus, where the union is not complete. If the sutures look like cutting out, they should be removed, and others put in their place. It is most important to get the gaping wound in the lid to heal with a broad soft scar; this is best achieved by frequent dabbing with a solution of silver nitrate, and by dressing with mild oils and ointments. When healing is complete the lids can be separated.

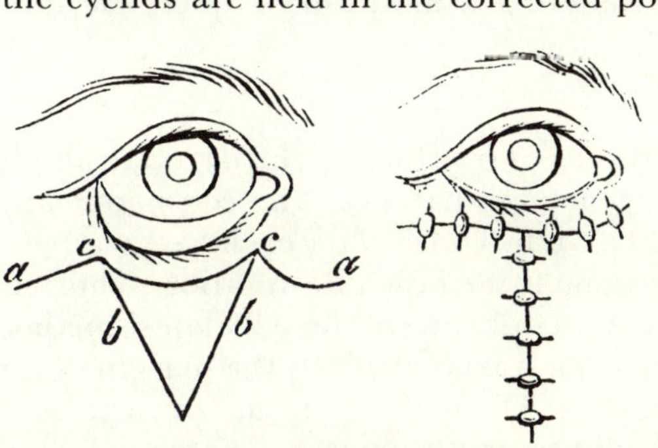

Fig. 30

Dieffenbach once said to me: 'there is not one of the many operations for ectropion that is the best; for some cases one method is preferable, for others another.' I certainly agree with this. His latest and most

[26] [See p. 96, n. 28.]

[27] [See n. 4 above.]

successful method gives such good results that it leaves hardly a trace. For the upper lid, he excises a triangle of skin at the outer canthus with its base about a quarter of an inch wide. Then he splits the outer commissure so that the incision runs into the base of this triangle. He frees the eyelid on its under-surface, and excises a strip of the tarsal margin (with its lashes) of the same length as the base of the triangle. This part of the lid is then drawn into the triangular defect at the angle, and fixed with fine insect-pins; the horizontal wound is closed with fine interrupted sutures. No raw surface is left. The operation is easier on the lower lid: the triangle is inverted, so that the base, where it is joined by the incision through the commissure, is uppermost. The great advantage of this method is that, even if primary healing does not occur, the contraction of the triangular wound will complete the cure.

Jäger's operation for lagophthalmos

This is not, as described by Dreyer,[28] a true blepharoplasty, but simply a plastic operation to cure lagophthalmos. In ectropion and lagophthalmos, both the height and the width of the eyelid are wrong—the first is too small, and the second is too large. Restoration to normal cannot be achieved by dealing with only one of these. Adams' method only reduces the width, by excising a triangle from the margin of the lid;[29] this leaves a contracting scar. Dieffenbach, in minor degrees of ectropion, excises a vertical ellipse to produce a lengthened scar. Jäger's operation is suitable for ectropion due to scarring, where the margin of the lid is stretched into a greater arc than normal (especially when the lid is adherent to the cheek or to the supraorbital margin), and also for severe lagophthalmos without eversion, or when a tumour has to be excised which leaves a small defect in the lid.

For several days before the operation, hard scars are softened, and the surrounding skin is stretched towards the eye with bandages. If the upper lid is adherent to the orbital margin, the eyebrow is shaved. Measurement with a thread will show how much longer the lid margin is than on the normal side.

The surgeon stands in front of the patient, holds the eyelid with forceps, and divides it horizontally in full thickness, *ab* [Fig. 31]. If he is afraid of damaging the eye, it can be protected by a horn spatula. A piece of tissue, *c*, is now excised in full thickness from this bridge; its width, determined by the previous measurement and marked out with

[28] [See n. 1 above.]

[29] [See n. 22 above.]

dye, is such as to make the two lid margins equal. Then, by a sawing action with a double-edged knife, the eyelid is freed from all adhesions, without exposing the bone. The two halves of the lid margin are joined with interrupted sutures, and the skin of the lid is then pulled down, and sutured horizontally; if the upper edge is too long, so that it makes a fold, this is excised. The sutures pick up the tarsus with the skin, but exclude the conjunctiva.

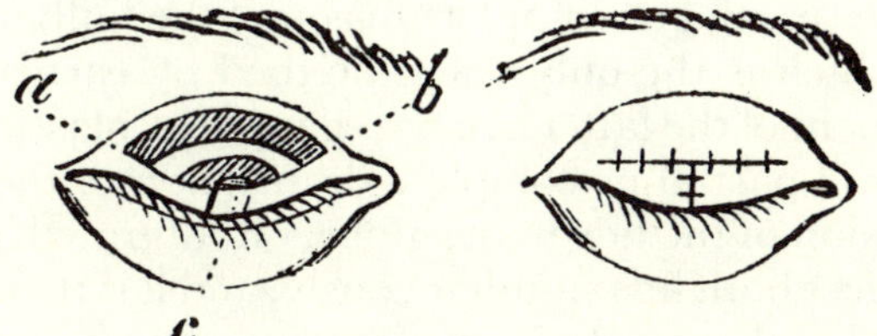

Fig. 31

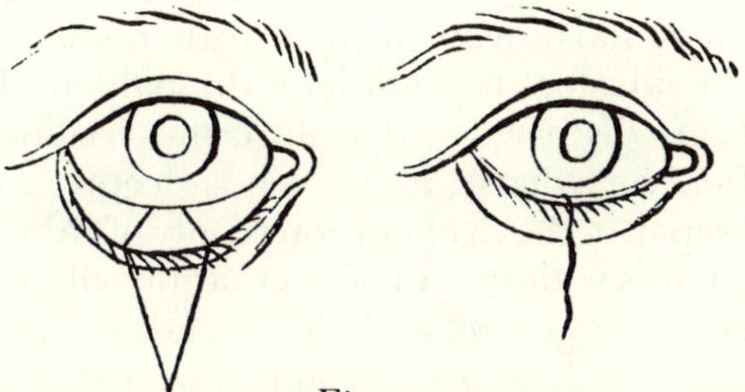

Fig. 32

For the lower lid, the same measurement is made and marked out, and continued down the cheek to form a triangle. One must also imagine two converging lines on the conjunctiva, because these cannot be marked [Fig. 32]. The whole segment is excised with a convex scalpel, through the full thickness of the eyelid, including the conjunctiva; the deeper tissues are divided with scissors curved on the flat. If necessary, the skin of the cheek is undermined to turn the lid in to the globe. Three or four twisted sutures are inserted; Jäger feels that these are not so suitable for the upper lid. The sutures are reinforced with English plaster,[30] and a compression bandage is used to push the skin towards the eyelid. The sutures are removed at 5–6 days, but the plaster should remain longer.

Case histories Two case histories in Dreyer's dissertation confirm the value of this method: a peasant's right upper eyelid had been damaged by erysipelas, so that he was left with such severe lagophthalmos that the centre of the lid margin was stuck to the bone. Apart from some pannus, the eye was healthy. The operation was successful, but it left a small coloboma, which was later excised and sutured. In the second case, a Hungarian girl had severe scarring of her face following burns when she rescued her old father from a fire. Her right lower eyelid was fixed to her cheek half an inch below the orbital margin. The left lower lid was less severely affected, but the eye had been destroyed. After

[30] [See p. 113, n. 15.]

bandaging to push the skin of the cheek towards the eye, the operation was successful.[31]

SYMBLEPHARON

Von Ammon has given a complete account of symblepharon.[32] He divides it into a posterior type (contraction of diseased conjunctiva where it passes from the globe to the lid), which is not part of plastic surgery, and an anterior type (partial or complete fusion of the bulbar conjunctiva with the lid), which is the only one described by earlier writers. His method of treatment of the latter can be regarded as plastic surgery. The condition follows partial or complete destruction of the conjunctiva, abnormal adhesion of the lids to the globe, or outgrowths on the conjunctiva. It may affect both lids simultaneously, and it is then often associated with ankyloblepharon. It is most common near the lacrimal punctum, and here it may be quite minor, usually following inflammation in the elderly, particularly women, with little disturbance of function. But when both sides or the middle of the palpebral opening are affected, the eyelids are distorted so that the lashes irritate the cornea. The adhesion is often very dense, and extends deeply, so that the tissues cannot easily be separated. An operation is only of value when the adhesion is small; when it is widespread, an operation will do harm by giving rise to profuse granulations and denser adhesions, which cannot be prevented by any medical or mechanical means.

Von Ammon's method for partial anterior symblepharon

The piece of the edge of the lid adherent to the globe is excised, leaving it in place, and the lid is repaired over it. Von Ammon had learned by bitter experience that simple separation of the adhesion is followed by recurrence, as the two raw surfaces stick together again. This gave him the idea of leaving tissue covered with skin on the surface of the eye. The eyelid is lifted on a probe, and two incisions are made with a cataract knife so that a triangular piece is left on the globe. If the gap in the lid is now too large to be sutured easily, the lid is undermined up to the orbital margin, as in Jäger's operation, until the skin is mobile enough. The two halves of the lid are then joined with three or four twisted sutures which include the tarsus. If there is still tension, a lateral incision, or dilatation of the palpebral opening, may be needed.

---

[31] [See n. 1 above.]

[32] F. A. von Ammon, *Das Symblepharon und die Heilung dieser Krankheit durch eine neue Operationsmethode*, 2nd edn, Dresden (1834).

The sutures are supported with sticking-plaster and a pressure bandage. The inner surface of the eyelid is now covered with healthy conjunctiva, which will not adhere to the epidermis on the piece of eyelid remaining on the globe. Any lashes on this piece must be plucked, and this is repeated as often as necessary.

In one of von Ammon's cases the epidermis began to look like mucous membrane after several weeks, and the piece became much smaller. If it irritates the lid or the eye, and particularly if there is any hope of improving vision, it can be excised when the lid has completely healed. After excision, the eye is irrigated with cold water every 2–3 hours, and later with lead lotion. The raw surface that is left is in contact with healthy conjunctiva, so that it will not adhere again. The granulations on the globe are treated with lead and zinc preparations, or dabbed with a solution of silver nitrate, to encourage healing.

Dieffenbach's method

If one or both eyelids are completely adherent, and there is a hope that there is only a superficial opacity in the cornea, Dieffenbach, for the lower lid, makes an incision from the inner canthus straight down to the border of the nose, and a second incision, of the same length, from the outer canthus to the infraorbital margin. The lid is held in fine forceps, and freed from the globe. This creates a square flap, attached only to the cheek. The eyelashes are shaved off. The lid is then turned in, so that its margin lies on the infra-orbital margin. Four or five sutures are inserted through this doubled lid, from without inwards, and then from within outwards, and tied on the skin. The globe cannot now become adherent, because the epidermal surface of the lid is turned towards it. When the globe has healed, this artificial entropion is opened out, and, with lateral incisions and insect-pins, the lid is restored to its old site. The globe is now covered with conjunctiva, and so it cannot adhere to the lid. The same technique is used for the upper lid, but both lids must not be operated on at the same time.[33]

ENTROPION

When entropion is due not only to laxity of the outer layers of the eyelid, but also, as is commonly the case, to distortion of the tarsal plate, the latter can be corrected by an operation that von Ammon calls '*tarsotomia longitudinalis*'.

---

33 Dieffenbach, *Erfahrungen*, Vol. 5 (1838) [unpublished].

Von Ammon's operation

The lid is transfixed, near the punctum, from within outwards with a double-bladed corneal knife, and incised parallel with, and about a quarter of an inch away from, the lid margin, ending one-third of an inch from the outer canthus. This incision is more easily made if the lid is supported on a horn spatula, as used in Jäger's operation. Sometimes such a long incision is not necessary, and a single puncture with the knife is enough. A piece of the skin of the lid is then excised with scissors in the usual way; when this is sutured, it holds the cut edges of the tarsal plate apart. An exudate forms in the gap, which not only restores the tarsal plate to its normal position, but also supports it, and prevents recurrence.

Brach's operation

Excision of tissue from the outside of the lid is not always successful in curing entropion, and the laxity of the skin leads to recurrence. Brach has therefore recommended a new technique. For either lid, a transverse incision, half an inch long, is made half an inch beyond the orbital margin. From the ends of this, two converging incisions end one-sixth of an inch from the lid margin [Fig. 33]. This flap is undermined, and as much is removed from its free end as has been determined by previous measurement; this is tested by advancing the flap, to bring the lid margin and the eyelashes into their normal position. The wound is sutured, and the eye is lightly bandaged for a few days to keep it still. The flap usually heals well. Brach thinks that this method can be used for most cases of entropion, whether due to shortening or to twisting of the tarsal plate; it can also be used for blepharoptosis and trichiasis. He has treated the lower lid of a girl aged 14, who had had a scrofulous infection for several years. Healing was so good that no trace of what had happened was to be seen.[34]

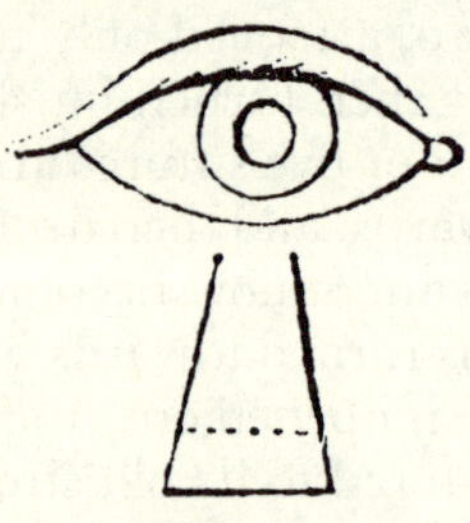

Fig. 33

[34] B. Brach, Vorschlag zu einer neuen Operationsmethode des Entropiums, *Preuss. med. Verztg.* p. 27 (1837).

13

LIP—CHEILOPLASTY

Cheiloplasty is the reconstruction of missing parts of the lip or the whole lip, and is thus quite different from the hare-lip operation, the cure of congenital or acquired clefts of the lip, and stomatoplasty. It is not a recent discovery, like blepharoplasty, for Tagliacozzi devoted a separate chapter to it.[1] His description was short, because most of the principles of rhinoplasty are applicable. Plastic operations are based on general principles, and anyone who wishes to carry out cheiloplasty must first know the rules for rhinoplasty.[2] Tagliacozzi divided deformed lips into congenital (hare-lip) and acquired. The operation for hare-lip is described in every surgical textbook, and will be omitted here. Congenital absence of the lip is unknown. The treatment of a hare-lip, even when the gap is very wide, or after removal of the central segment in a double cleft, does not need transplantation of a flap, for the two halves of the lip can always be drawn together. Many diseases of the upper lip, or the reconstruction of the columella, may require the excision of a triangular piece of the lip, and this can be repaired exactly as a hare-lip. But this is still very different from a true cheiloplasty. It is a common mistake nowadays to use this term for simple repair of the lip.

Acquired defects are commonly due to cancer, mostly in the lower lip. In the upper lip this hardly ever occurs unless a spongy tumour or a chancre has turned into cancer, or a true cancer has spread from the angle of the mouth or the ala. Other causes can, of course, affect either lip. Prisoners of war in India are said to have their lips, as well as their noses and ears, cut off. With us, destruction of the lips sometimes results from suicidal attempts. In childhood, noma can destroy the lips completely, and, as Roux has pointed out, the lack of counter-pressure from the soft tissues may lead to asymmetrical development of the jaws. In one case, before he could reconstruct the lip, he had to resect part of

---

[1] Tagliacozzi, *de curtorum,* Vol. 2. Chapter 19.

[2] 'We would advise surgeons that they are not competent to graft lips unless they have thoroughly mastered the restoration of noses, and have tested their skill in this. For the other operations are derived from it, as rivers from a source; they are its seeds, and they cannot equal it, for it is the pre-eminent operation.' (ibid, p. 67).

the mandible.[3] Burns produce adhesion of the lips to each other and to the jaws, rather than complete destruction.

THE ITALIAN METHOD

Tagliacozzi reconstructed lips, like the nose, from the arm. But he warned against the operation, unless it was absolutely necessary. It is less successful than rhinoplasty, because the flow of saliva and mucus interferes with healing. The rules for the preparation of the flap are the same as for rhinoplasty, with careful measurement of the size of the defect. For the lower lip, the pedicle must be at the upper end near the shoulder, so that the flap is not twisted; to attach it to the lip, it is turned over and sutured with its raw surface uppermost. In 1819, Gräfe used the Italian method, following Tagliacozzi's instructions exactly.

Case-report A weaver aged 21 had lost his upper lip and part of the cheek from gangrene following typhus. The surrounding tissues were densely scarred. On 13 December 1819 the flap was raised as a bridge six inches long and three inches wide. There was a profuse discharge of pus, needing dressings twice a day. The flap contracted, and after three weeks its under-surface was covered with epidermis. The upper transverse incision was therefore made on 6 January 1820. The flap rapidly shrank and went pale; after several days the colour returned. The attachment to the lip was made on 4 February, and the arm was fixed in the harness. By the seventh day the flap was firmly united, and it was separated from the arm. At first it survived well, but it then became gangrenous and was lost.[4]

This case has already been discussed because of its physiological interest.[5]

THE INDIAN METHOD

The Indian surgeon who carried out Cowasjee's rhinoplasty in Poona could also restore lips, 'and wanted to perform that operation on the eldest son of our native ambassador at the Paishwah's court, who had lost part of his upper lip: but to this he would not agree, although they told him that they had frequently done it with success.'[6] Lynn[7] and

---

3 [See n. 27 below.]

4 C. F. von Gräfe, Neue Beiträge, p. 10 (1821).

5 See p. 70.

6 Letter from Colonel J. Ward, 12 November 1815 to Carpue. In *Two successful operations*, p, 102.

7 [W. Lynn. In C. Bell, *Institutes of Surgery*, Vol. 1, Edinburgh, p. 226 (1838).]

Sutcliffe[8] in England carried out reconstruction of the lip by the Indian method. Boyer reported that Chopart had operated in the Indian manner for cancer of the lip with skin from the neck.[9] Malgaigne describes simple suture of the lip as '*procédé de Chopart*'.[10]

Delpech, after several rhinoplastic operations, carried out a cheiloplasty in 1823, which he called '*l'achyloplastique*'.[11] The derivation of this term is hard to guess, but it is a worthy counterpart to Richerand's '*rhymnoplastique*' and Labat's '*rhytnomètes*'. However, Delpech is a better surgeon than etymologist, and his operation shows that he has a talent for this type of surgery. His experience led him to prefer the Indian to the Italian method, but he is wrong in thinking that his is the only method. His cheiloplasty was one of the earliest since the resurgence of plastic surgery in Europe. It failed almost completely, although this seems to have been due more to faulty technique, for it was based on correct principles, which, with some modification, should give successful results.

Case-report A man aged 54 had had nearly the whole of his lower lip destroyed by cancer, leaving only small remnants at the angles of the mouth. The tumour extended to the chin. The gum was involved, but mobile, so that the bone appeared to be unaffected. It would therefore be possible to remove all diseased tissue, leaving the bone intact, and leaving part of the muscle to give some movement to the reconstructed lip. There were no enlarged glands. Delpech decided to take the skin from below the chin, as it was healthy and mobile. He was afraid that a simple flap would adhere to the gum at its upper end, and this gave him the idea of doubling over the upper part of the flap, reckoning from previous experience that constant contact with saliva would make the skin like mucous membrane. He drew the pattern on the skin of the neck, leaving a pedicle one and a half inches wide [Fig. 34]. After excising the tumour with the gum, he raised the flap, and cut off the tip which had only been included to make suture of the neck easier. The distal third of the flap was doubled over and fixed to the middle third with two sutures. Then the flap was brought up into position, and sutured to the sides of the lip. The wound in the neck, extending to the

---

8 [Carpue, *Two successful operations, p. 40.*]

9 A. Boyer, Mémoire sur la meilleure forme des aiguilles propres à la réunion des plaies, *Mém. soc. méd. émul.* p. 97. (Paris, 1799). [See also: J. Thomson, *Lectures on inflammation,* Edinburgh, p. 230 (1813).]

10 J. F. Malgaigne, *Manuel de médecine opératoire,* Brussels, p. 462 (1834).

11 J. M. Delpech, *Chirurgie clinique,* Vol. 2, p. 587.

sternum, was sutured. The patient was not unduly affected by the operation, but on the fourth day a foul smell indicated that the inner layer of the flap was dead. Over the next few days the greater part of the rest of the flap became gangrenous.

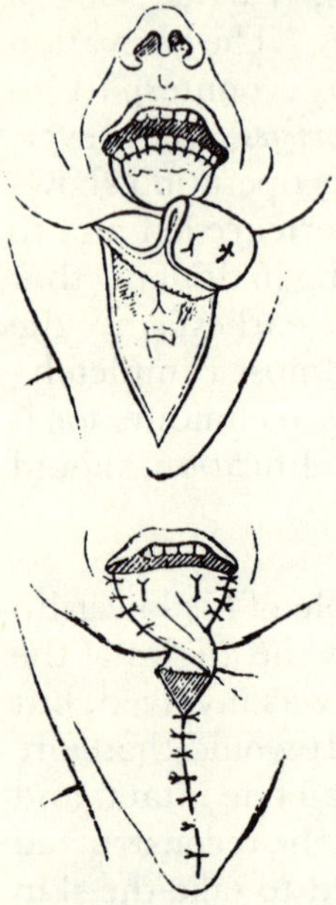

Fig. 34

Dupuytren also transplanted skin from the neck, in three stages, for a child who had lost the commissure, part of the upper lip, and the greater part of the right side of the mandible from gangrene.[12]

The study of cheiloplasty is made very difficult by the number of operative methods, named after different surgeons by different authors, which all seem to be more or less the same. Velpeau says of cheiloplasty: 'it is an operation that cannot be subjected to detailed rules; it must be modified almost every time it is done'. Here only the important and general differences, and not the minor modifications, will be discussed. The Italian method can be used for the upper or the lower lip, and the Indian method, from the neck, for the lower. Textor[13] and Lallemand[14], have used the latter to replace the lower lip , and part of the cheek.

The tendency of the flap to contract, or to adhere to the jaw, and the poor resemblance to a normal lip, have led many surgeons to retain the lateral parts (for the upper lip as well as the lower), and simply to draw them together. I had a successful case in a small child with a *naevus maternus*[15] of the greater part of the upper lip, which looked like a turkey's comb. I had to remove most of the upper lip and columella, but, after freeing the mucous membrane from the upper jaw, I was able to join the remaining segments with hare-lip sutures. Healing was excellent by the seventh day, when the last of the sutures were removed and replaced with sticking-plaster. But the wet-nurse, against my instructions, put the child back on the breast, and the wound broke down. I re-sutured it, and it healed so well that there was only a linear scar to be seen.

---

[12] G. Dupuytren, Chéiléoplastie, pratiquée avec succès, *Gaz. Höp. Paris*, p. 273 (1830).

[13] K. Textor, Ueber Chiloplastik', *Isis*, **21**, 496 (1828).

[14] C.-F. Lallemand, Plaie à la face avec perte de substance, guérie par l'application d'un lambeau détaché des parties voisines, *Archs gén. Méd.* **6**, 242 (1824).

[15] [Haemangioma.]

Many operations of this sort have been described as reconstructions of the lip: Chelius for the upper lip,[16] Riberi,[17] Berg,[18] and several by Dieffenbach,[19] who sometimes freed the soft tissues as far as the masseter in order to be able to bring them together. Dupuytren went even further than this, by dividing part of the cheek to move it into a defect of the lower lip.

Case-report A man aged 36 had lost part of his mandible, most of the lower lip, and the soft tissues down to the hyoid from a self-inflicted gunshot wound. This healed in two months, but contracture of the remaining muscles had pulled the fragment of mandible up to the level of the ala. Dupuytren operated on 16 April 1831, exposing and sawing off the displaced bone. An incision dividing the cheek for one and a half inches allowed the remaining ends of the lower lip to be united. The lower part of the wound was sutured after the scarred edges had been excised. Some parts of the wound granulated, but treatment by cauterization, sticking-plaster, and compression brought about almost complete healing in two months. The patient was left with only linear scars instead of a large hole into his mouth. The lower jaw was missing, but there is no way on earth of replacing this.[20]

Dieffenbach introduced an ingenious modification by using part of the upper lip to replace the lower.

Case-report A man aged 60 had had a carcinoma of the lower lip for several years, which had destroyed the whole lip from the angles of the mouth down to the chin. His upper lip was unusually large, so that one could have made two lips out of it. The patient had undergone the Zittmann treatment[21] for several weeks. When he was somewhat recovered, Dieffenbach operated on him, excising the whole handful of cauliflower-like tumour from the angles of the mouth down to two inches below the chin. The periosteum of the mandible was considerably thickened. He freed the cheek back to the masseter, and separated it from the whole lower border of the mandible. After controlling the

---

[16] M. J. Chelius, Gelungene Lippen- und Nasenbilding an demselben Subjecte, *Heidelb. klin. Annln.* **6,** 523 (1830).

[17] A. Riberi, Fall von Lippenbildung, *Repert. med. chir, Piemonte* (Oct. 1834).

[18] Berg, Chiloplastik, *Preuss. med. Verztg.* p. 251 (1836).

[19] Dieffenbach, *Erfahrungen,* Vol. 3, p. 96 (1834).

[20] Dupuytren, *Leçons orales,* Vol. 1, p. 25 (1832).

[21] [See p. 61, n. 11.]

severe bleeding, he cauterized the diseased periosteum with a red-hot iron. Then he made an oblique incision in the upper lip for one inch from each angle of the mouth nearly up to the columella. This made two pointed flaps which were to form part of the lower lip. In spite of pulling strongly on sutures through the cheeks a gap of one inch remained. He therefore made a relieving incision two inches long in each cheek, half-way between the edge of the wound and the anterior border of the masseter, and large enough to take two fingers. This enabled the wound to be closed without tension. Finally, the flaps from the upper lip were turned down with their tips together, so that the new lower lip, made from the cheek, was covered with red margin from the upper lip. The patient's appearance was now quite tolerable, except that, if he opened his mouth, you could see right across, as if a bullet had passed through it, for the tension had made the lateral incisions almost circular. Suppuration only occurred in two places; the tips of the flaps healed well. The lateral openings closed spontaneously in four weeks without leaving a fistula. His mouth was, for a man, rather small, but it looked quite natural, with proper angles and a lower lip with a red margin.

Dieffenbach now repairs large losses of the lower lip with incisions outwards from the angles of the mouth, and then downwards (see Fig. 35), to make two flaps, which are brought together in the midline and covered with mucous membrane. Previously he used to resect the chin in order to get enough soft tissue.

Chopart's method

Chopart's method, as it is called by Velpeau, Malgaigne, van Es, and others, is nothing more than advancement of skin from the chin. This is always unsatisfactory, as the flap is too short. Chopart excised the tumour through vertical incisions from the angles of the mouth, down to a little way below the chin, joined by a curved transverse incision. The vertical incisions extended beyond the transverse incision to make a square flap, which was simply advanced and sutured to the cheeks. This flap will naturally tend to retract, especially in the middle. Cambrelin described a similar operation.[22]

Richerand's method

This is even less effective: the tumour is excised with scissors, and the mucous membrane is divided where the lip meets the gum, to allow the

[22] Cambrelin, Chéiléoplastie, *Archs gén. Méd.* **26,** 263 (1831).

skin to be advanced and held with bandages and plaster. This is not much better than simple excision and leaving the defect to close by scar-tissue.[23]

Roux de St. Maximin's method

This method, with which Velpeau is said to have got very good results,[24] is nearly the same: the skin over the mandible and upper part of the neck is undermined, pulled over the defect like an apron, and held with sticking-plaster. If the angles of the mouth have to be extended by horizontal incisions, the apron is sutured to the upper lip. The patient's head has to be kept firmly flexed until healing is complete. This is not only tiresome for the surgeon, who has to adjust the fixation, but very hard on the patient. This would be no criticism of the operation if it was justified by the results, which is not the case. Blandin used the same technique.[25] Serre, in Montpellier, altered this by keeping the healthy tissue from the lip for lining, which he sutured to the flap from the cheek.[26]

Roux's method

This method, as described by Maisonabe,[27] and Velpeau,[28] is unusual in that part of an over-prominent chin was sawn off to make repair of the lip easier.

Case report A woman had lost all but a small piece of the right side of both lips in childhood. The deformity was made worse by the prominence of the mandible, which was due to its growth unrestrained by the lips. Roux removed an inch of bone from the enlarged mandible, and the soft tissues then came together easily. Some weeks later he wanted to operate on the upper jaw in the same way, but the patient refused.

The powerful influence of the soft tissues on the development of bone has, up to now, had too little attention paid to it. Imperfectly formed

[23] A.-B. Richerand, *Nosographie et thérapeutique chirugicales*, 5th edn, Vol. 4, Paris, p. 341 (1821).

[24] A. L. M. Velpeau, *Nouveaux éléments de médecine opératoire*, Vol. 2, Paris, p. 33 (1832).

[25] P. F. Blandin, Autoplastie faciale, *Bull, Acad. r. Méd.* **1,** 34 (1836).

[26] M. Serre, Nouveau procédé de chéiloplastie, *Gaz. Méd.* p. 238 (1835).

[27] C. A. Maisonabe, *Clinique sur les difformités dans l'espèce humaine*, Vol. 2 Paris, p. 97 (1834).

[28] See n. 24 above.

bones may return, at least partly, to normal when the soft tissues are restored. Bony clefts will become narrower, and may even fuse, as after the repair of a cleft palate.

The above examples show that many of the operations dignified by the name of 'cheiloplasty' are little better than what used to be called 'the operation for cancer of the lip', where there was no plastic surgery, and the skin was simply drawn together with plaster. These operations leave the teeth uncovered, and the two lips are not in contact; they do not deserve to be called 'cheiloplasty'. Some of the methods are suitable for small defects, but in many cases there is not enough local skin. It is a disadvantage to have to take the skin from the face, and a large flap from the neck leaves an ugly contracted scar that restricts movement. The great difficulty in reconstructing the lip is that it consists, like the eyelid, of two surfaces, of which the posterior must be covered with mucous membrane to prevent it becoming adherent to the gum. Serre tried to solve this by saving as much as possible of the mucous membrane of the old lip to line the back of the new lip.[29] But the tissue must be healthy, and, even then, it does not always heal as well as could be wished. In other cases there is nothing left of the lip to be saved. Another complication is the immobility of the new lip. Only when part of the old lip is present can the new lip regain even a little movement. However, a reconstructed lip serves to improve the appearance, to prevent dribbling, blackening and falling-out of the teeth, and prolapse of the tongue; sometimes speech is improved, and chewing is made easier.

Dieffenbach's method

Cheiloplasty would be in a poor way if there was nothing better than has been described so far. But, like all other plastic operations, it blossomed as soon as Dieffenbach took it up. He developed it in two ways: firstly, by using relieving incisions (which he had reintroduced into surgery), carried out with his usual boldness, incising not only the skin but the full thickness of the cheeks; and secondly, as with blepharoplasty, by introducing the transposed flap, and making the new lip not only of skin, but of the full thickness of the cheeks. Rost described the first of these in his dissertation.[30]

Case-report A man aged 49 with an extensive carcinoma of the lower lip, chin, and parts of the cheeks was admitted to the Charité in Berlin.

---

[29] [See n. 26 above.]

[30] G. Rost, *De chilo- et stomatoplastice*, Diss., Berlin, p. 22 (1836).

The tumour was adherent to the mandible, but there were no enlarged glands. Dieffenbach excised the whole mass with the involved periosteum and the lower border of the mandible. Bleeding was very severe—all the vessels seemed to be enlarged. The defect was more than a handsbreadth. In order to slacken the tissues, the upper lip was freed from the maxilla as far back as the masseter. But when the edges of the wound were pulled together as hard as possible there was still a gap of three inches. Dieffenbach therefore made relieving incisions in the cheeks, from the zygoma down to the border of the mandible, in full thickness; they were so large that three or four fingers could be inserted. This allowed the wound edges to be closed in the midline with long insect-pins. The lateral openings were dressed with lint to keep out the air, and an ice-bag was placed on the lower half of the face. The next day the patient was very well. There was marked swelling and redness; 30 leeches were applied. At eight days, two-thirds of the wound had healed by first intention. The upper part suppurated, and was held together with sticking-plaster. The right lateral opening was dry, but saliva was still coming from the left. When everything was nearly completely healed a recurrence was noticed. A red-hot iron was applied, Zittmann's decoction[31] was given by mouth, and the patient was discharged from hospital.

Dieffenbach's second method

This is quite different. Instead of pulling the cheeks together, it is a true reconstruction of the lip, not only with skin, but also with muscle and mucous membrane. The idea came to him at the same time as his reconstruction of the eyelid by skin from the temple.[32] He decided to use the scar contracture of the secondary defects to keep the new lip stretched out flat. After excising the tumour, or freshening the margins of the defect, he makes horizontal incisions, 1–2 inches long, from the angles of the mouth through the cheeks, *ab* [Fig. 35]. The combined length of these incisions should be slightly greater than the width of the upper lip. From the ends of these,

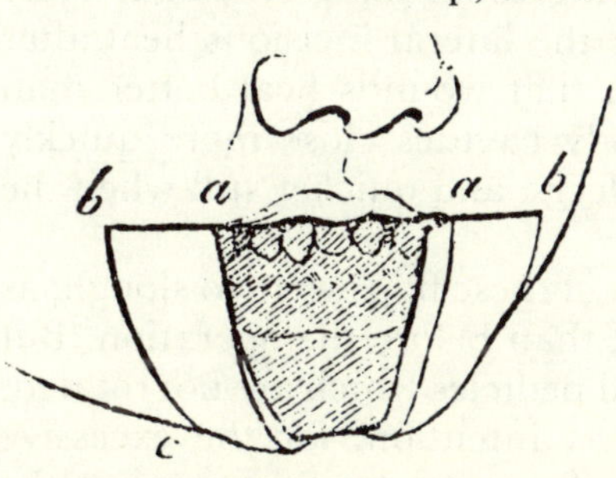

Fig. 35

[31] [See p. 61, n. 11.]

[32] See p. 137, n. 11.

two vertical incisions, *bc*, also in full thickness, run downwards and slightly forwards to the lower border of the mandible, or further if necessary. Thus a flap is formed on each side of the defect, with a pedicle more than one inch wide at the lower border of the mandible. To make the flaps more mobile the mucous membrane is divided where it passes on to the gum. It must be admitted that the raising of such flaps in full thickness is a traumatic procedure.

The internal maxillary artery must be ligated where it crosses the border of the mandible, and before it has given off the coronary artery to the lower lip, but this does not endanger the blood-supply of the flaps. There is also the risk of cutting Stensen's duct in the vertical incision, which leads to a temporary salivary fistula. The mucosa on each flap is now joined to the skin with interrupted sutures to make the red margin of the lip. The flaps are brought into the midline and sutured with insect-pins [Fig. 36].

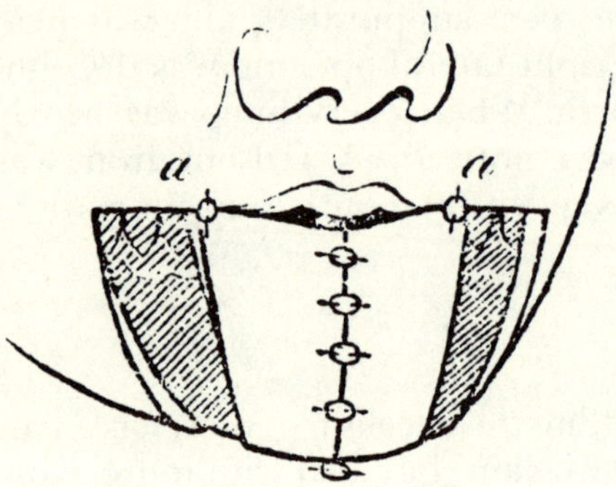

Fig. 36

One suture at each corner of the mouth (*a,a*) holds the flaps up; this was the reason for making the horizontal incisions wider than the upper lip. The new lip is lined with mucosa, so that it cannot become adherent to the gum. The lateral defects will leak saliva at first, but granulations and the flexibility of the soft tissues will bring about complete closure, just as the lateral incisions heal after repair of the palate. It is well known that wounds heal better than ulcers, and that perforations into body cavities close more quickly when they are due to injury than to ulcers, and quicker still when the injury is not accidental, but surgical.

It would be disastrous if one or both of these flaps were to slough, as this would leave the patient worse off than before the operation. But this is unlikely, as they have very broad pedicles which are not rotated. They can be expected to heal by first intention, for the excessive inflammation that most commonly interferes with healing occurs in the skin to which a flap is attached. But this does not happen when the cut edges of two flaps are apposed, for they readily adhere by agglutination. This is due to the lowered vitality of flaps, which is particularly favourable for primary healing. The most that is to be feared from this operation is that the tips of the flaps may not heal to the angles of the mouth. For this reason the patient must not try to open his mouth, and the new lip must be supported with sticking-plaster. If these areas break down they should at once be re-sutured, so that the flaps do not retract. Touching with silver nitrate, or small relieving incisions, will encourage the lateral incisions to close.

In cases where the mandible is stripped of its soft tissues Dieffenbach resects the bone to allow the edges to come together, for a length of bone that has been laid bare will die.

Blasius' operation

Blasius has described a new technique, somewhat similar to Dieffenbach's, which is one of the best methods of lip reconstruction. Only the skin is used, instead of the full thickness of the cheeks.[33]

Case-report Blasius excised the whole lower lip, in a man aged 55, going beyond the angle of the mouth on the right side *a*, including all the soft tissues of the chin, and continuing the incisions down to half an inch below the mandible, *b* [Fig. 37]. The bone was exposed in several places; one discoloured area was shaved off. Spurting arteries were twisted off, so that no ligatures would be left in the wound to delay healing. From each edge of the wound a second incision at right angles, starting half an inch above the lower border of the mandible, was made downwards for a good inch, and then curving up along the jaw to the masseter *c*. On the left side, the incision started further from the jaw, so that the flap was shorter. The two cheek flaps were undermined, and their narrow ends were sutured together with insect-pins (*a,a*) [Fig. 38]. The corners (*b,b*) were then undermined, and, with the head flexed, sutured to each other and to the lower

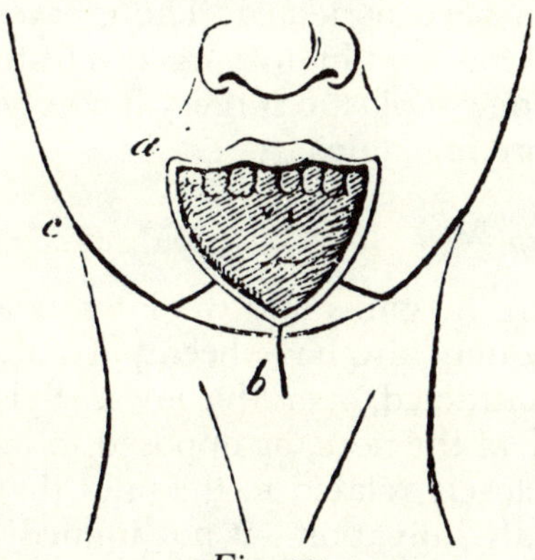

Fig. 37

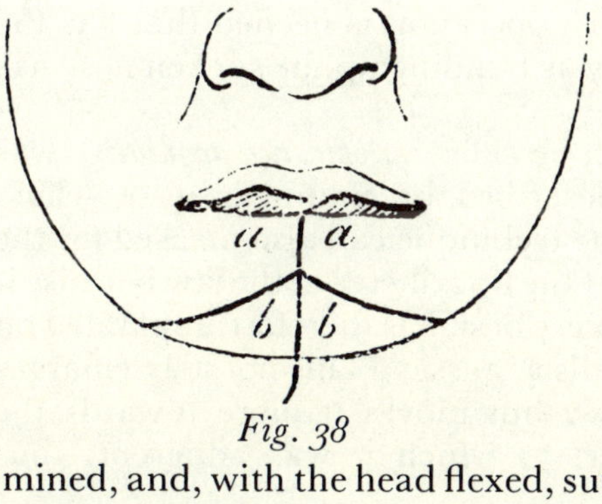

Fig. 38

[33] E. Blasius, Neues Verfahren der Lippenbildung, *Z. Chir, Augenheilk.* **1,** p. 387 (1836).

margins of the cheek flaps. No dressing was used, but the wound was covered with a cold wet cloth which the patient held between his teeth; his head was kept flexed. With frequent cold compresses the wound mostly healed by first intention, but the free border granulated, and he was left with a narrow band of scar between the mucosa and the skin—as seen after crescentic excisions for cancer. The new lip contracted a little, so that the lower teeth were not completely covered, but it could still meet the upper lip.

Blasius intends to reconstruct the upper lip in the same way when a suitable patient presents. Two cheek flaps, or one if only half the lip is missing, would be turned up under the nose, and the secondary defects would be sutured. Experience is needed to show whether this is practicable. Similarly, other methods for the lower lip might be modified and used for the upper lip. But reconstruction is needed much more often for the lower lip, so that this has been perfected. The greater difficulty of reconstructing the upper lip has kept many surgeons from attempting it, but with growing knowledge of plastic surgery it can be expected that surgeons will become more ingenious.

Von Ammon's operation for adhesion of the lip

The lips commonly become adherent to the gums and the jaws as a result of treatment with mercury. They may also have been partially destroyed, or have become tightly contracted over the jaws. This condition may be compared to collapse of the nose, as opposed to its complete destruction. The lips are so closely related to the jaws that adhesion must always follow [mercurial] salivation—if not immediately, then later. Cutting the lips free from the jaw is useless, for the adhesion always quickly recurs. An operation is needed that has the same relation to a true cheiloplasty as building up the sunken nose has to a full rhinoplasty.

Von Ammon's operation, which he calls '*chiloplastica angularis*', was used by him in two cases (as described by Baumgarten[34]), which involved the upper lip only, but the technique can also be used for the lower lip. It is based on the fact that the lip adheres to the jaw because it is so tightly stretched across it. A piece of skin is therefore implanted on each side—what the seamstress calls a 'gusset'. This not only enlarges and slackens the lip over the jaw, but moves it more towards the midline, and away from the part to which it was adherent, thus preventing recurrence.

---

[34] M. Baumgarten, *De chiloplastica et stomatopoësi*, Leipzig, p. 46 (1837).

Von Ammon divides all adhesions between the lip and the jaw, and then cuts through the full thickness of the lip near the angle of the mouth, creating a gaping triangular defect with its short side towards the lower lip. This is done on both sides of the mouth, otherwise the lip will become asymmetrical [Fig. 39]. It is important to extend the incision out into the cheek for half an inch, so that the flap is not raised too near the mouth, where a scar might produce further tension in the lip. The outline of the flap is then drawn on the cheek as a triangle which should be slightly larger than the defect, leaving a narrow pedicle, *ad*, about a quarter of an inch wide. The smaller triangle, *ceb*, is excised after the flap has been raised, so that the wound in the cheek is easier to close. The pattern is tested to make sure that the flap will be the right size. The flap is then raised and turned into the defect; this is easy, as it only has to be turned through 90°. Suturing starts at the margin of the lip; near the pedicle there is not enough room for twisted sutures, and interrupted sutures are used. Finally, the horizontal wound is easily closed. The sutures nearest the margin of the lip are removed last.

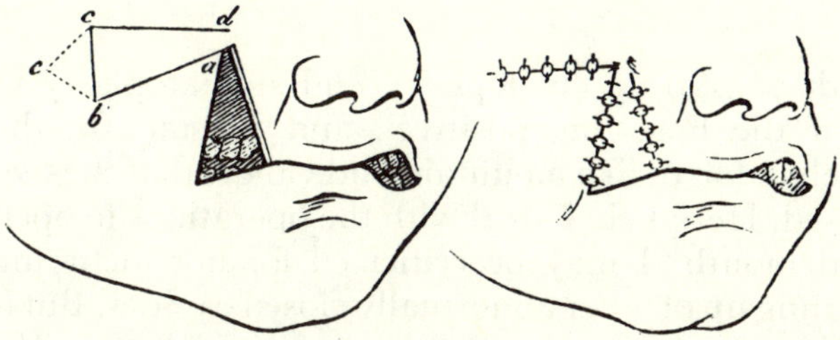

Fig. 39

After carrying out this operation in selected cases it is encouraging to find that the adhesion does not recur. This is all the more valuable, as the earlier methods usually consisted of the insertion of lead plates, or other foreign material, which were not tolerated by the patient or, if they were, were almost never successful.

14
MOUTH—STOMATOPLASTY

No apology is needed for putting cheiloplasty and stomatoplasty in separate chapters, for the lips, the 'positive', and the mouth, the 'negative', are so closely related, like mountain and valley, that the two terms are often confused. Here I shall deal with the operations to open an abnormally closed mouth. I may be criticized for not including operations for the opening up of other abnormally closed cavities. But it is the technique of the operation, and not its purpose, that makes stomatoplasty part of plastic surgery, as well as its relation to reconstruction of the lip.

CONTRACTURE OF THE MOUTH

Closure of the mouth by scar-tissue is one of the most terrible deformities of the human face. It commonly follows syphilitic and phagedaenic ulcers, and, sometimes, heavy doses of mercury or *herpes rodens*.[1] The patient has a hole the size of a finger instead of a mouth. This gradually contracts further until it is difficult to get fluids in. Some of these poor wretches die of hunger; others survive by stuffing small bits of food in with their fingers, and sucking fluids through a quill. The tissues round the mouth are very rigid, so that chewing is difficult, and digestion is upset. There is great discomfort from the masses of tartar that cover the teeth. A strong jet of foul breath comes out of the mouth, especially when the nose has collapsed and the nostrils are obstructed.

Dieffenbach describes three types of contracture:

1. The inner surfaces of the lips and cheeks are adherent to the jaws, but the skin is relatively undamaged; this occurs in children who have been given a lot of calomel.
2. The lips are adherent to each other, and the mouth is converted into a round hole; this sometimes follows severe burns or *herpes exedens*.[2]

---

[1] [See p. 53, n. 1.]
[2] [See p. 53, n. 1.]

3. The outer parts of the lips are destroyed, together with the surrounding tissues, so that the teeth are exposed, and the jaws cannot be separated; occasionally the mouth opens on to the cheek.

All three types are common following the overuse of mercury.[3]

Earlier treatment

This consisted of dilatation with bougies or tents (very uncomfortable for the patient), simple incision, or the insertion of foreign bodies in the angles of the mouth, which caused such a severe reaction that they all had to be removed. None of these did any good, for the contracture always rapidly recurred. Krüger-Hansen treated a girl whose mouth was closed on the left side, as a result of smallpox, so that she could only get a small teaspoon in. He pushed a trocar through the place where the angle of the mouth should have been, and left a lead wire in the track until this was established, which he encouraged with silver nitrate dissolved in lead lotion. Then he cut away the superfluous tissue. This healed well, but the lip did not regain its proper shape because the mouth was surrounded by scar.[4]

This is the same principle as Rudtorffer's treatment of fused fingers.[5]

Dieffenbach's treatment

Dieffenbach found that this method either did not succeed at all, or it took six months for the track to become established; sometimes the wire became displaced or it cut through. He discovered a quicker and surer method by covering the cut edges with mucous membrane. He described this first in 1827,[6] and in more detail in 1829,[7] particularly for use in his second group, where the two lips are fused together.

Case report In a contracture of the mouth following *herpes exedens*, Dieffenbach pushed the pointed blade of a pair of sharp scissors into the upper corner of one side of the opening, between the soft tissues of the

[3] Dieffenbach, *Erfahrungen*, Vol. 3, p. 66 (1834).

[4] B. K. Krüger-Hansen, Practische Reminiscenzen, *J. Chir. Augenheilk.* **4**, 543 (1822).

[5] F. X. Rudtorffer, *Abhandlung über die einfachste und sicherste Operationsmethode eingesperrter Leisten- und Schenkelbrüche*, Vol. 2, Vienna, p. 453 (1808).

[6] Dieffenbach, Neue Methode der Lippenbildung, *Magazin ges. Heilk.* **25**, 383 (1827).

[7] Dieffenbach, *Erfahrungen*, Vol. 1, p. 44 (1829).

cheek and the mucous membrane, and divided the former. He could then get his finger into the opening. Holding the cheek forwards, he pushed the blade further, and divided the outer layers up to the point where he intended to make the angle of the mouth. He made a similar incision from the lower corner, parallel to the first, joining them by a short curved incision at the angle. He then excised the intervening strip of skin, and repeated the procedure on the other side of the mouth. The patient could now open his mouth, separating the wound edges widely, so that the retained mucous membrane was stretched out like a web. This was incised, advanced, and sutured around the mouth, and into the angles, with interrupted and twisted sutures, as the edge of a shoe is oversewn with its lining. It healed completely, and the patient was left with not merely an opening, but a real mouth with red lips.

Since then Dieffenbach has often used this method with great success, frequently for fusion of one angle of the mouth, or after excision of cancer of the lip involving the angle.

For the treatment of the first type, where the lips are adherent to the jaws,[8] all strands of scar-tissue are divided; posteriorly this is better done with scissors. At intervals the patient should be allowed to wash his mouth out thoroughly with water. If the adhesion is only due to strands of scar it will be healed in a few days. If there is adhesion of a whole surface, undamaged mucosa is undermined to the thickness of cardboard, pulled over the raw surface, and held with interrupted sutures; the posterior sutures can be inserted with a fine perforated hook. Dieffenbach treated seven patients successfully by this method, although one of them died of mercurial cachexia.

In the third type, where parts of the lips have been destroyed, more of a reconstructive operation is needed. There are no general rules for this, and each case must be left to the decision of the surgeon. A detailed plan must be made beforehand, so that, if the operation is likely to prove too traumatic, it can be divided into several stages. Here is an example of Dieffenbach's great talent for devising the most appropriate operation for a frightful deformity:

Case report A 19-year-old bookseller had no mouth or lips, but on his right cheek was a hole the size of a hen's egg, with its margin fused to the gum in a cartilaginous mass; the surrounding tissues were grossly scarred. He could not open his teeth even a hair's breadth, and could

[8] [See also p. 160.]

only suck in fluids through a raven's quill. The operation was one of the bloodiest that could be imagined. Dieffenbach began by trying to close the opening in the cheek by excising the surrounding scars and separating the soft tissues from the upper and lower jaws. Then he cut with scissors into the place where the mouth should be. Through this opening he freed further adhesions until the jaws could be separated, and the mouth cleared of concretions. Unfortunately there was very little mucous membrane left on the cheeks to be used in the repair. The defect in the cheek was now sutured, but there was so much tension that a relieving incision was made along the anterior border of the masseter. Bleeding here was unusually heavy, but it was controlled with cold water.

The poor young man withstood this fearful operation with exemplary courage, only letting out an occasional groan. He was put back to bed, on a cooling regime, with an ice-bag on his face and a syringe for him to squirt cold water into his mouth. Fever was slight, and he thought himself lucky to be able to take large draughts of cold water. The swelling was no greater than expected, and all the sutures were removed on the third day. Only half the wound healed, but, as there was no tension, the edges could be held together with sticking-plaster. After six weeks, scar-contracture round the new mouth prevented him separating his teeth. Dieffenbach divided the new adhesions, and turned in a small skin flap to establish the angle of the mouth. Several further small operations were carried out to improve the appearance of the lips by giving them a red margin.[9]

Werneck's treatment

Werneck announced that, in 1817, he had already transplanted mucous membrane for contraction of the mouth, but he did not publish this until after Dieffenbach had described his method of lining reconstructed lips.[10] Werneck's technique is only suitable for cases where the mucosa is undamaged.

Case reports A pensioner aged 35 had severe contracture of his mouth following syphilitic herpes. In 1817, Werneck incised both sides of the mouth, so that he could get a finger in. He excised an ellipse of scar on each side, and divided all tissues including the orbicularis. The mucous

---

[9] Dieffenbach, *Erfahrungen*, Vol. 3, p. 110 (1834).

[10] W. Werneck, Ueber die künstliche Mundwinkel- und Lippenbildung durch blütige Umschlagung der Mundschleimhaut, *J. Chir. Augenheilk.* **14**, 202 (1830).

membrane was then freed from the muscle, stretched to cover the raw surfaces, and attached by interrupted sutures to line the angles of the mouth. Four hours after the operation, when the exudate had stopped, Werneck covered the sutures with gold-beater's skin.[11] The patient was forbidden to talk for 10 days, and was fed on soup from a cup with a spout. Healing was then complete, and he was able to open his mouth freely from then on.

The second case was a girl aged 16 with severe scarring of both angles of her mouth and destruction of the centre of both lips, so that her teeth were exposed. There were also adhesions restricting the movements of her jaw. Werneck enlarged the mouth and divided the adhesions. The mucosa of the lips was hard and scarred, and he therefore used the mucosa of the cheeks from the region of the molar teeth to line the angles of the mouth.

The third patient was an officer's servant, who had shot himself, but survived with his face almost split in two. As it healed his mouth became increasingly contracted. Several attempts by Rudtorffer's method failed.[12] Werneck raised a narrow triangular flap on the cheek, with its tip at the point where the angle of the mouth should be. He detached the mucosa and muscle, turned the flap in, and fixed it by passing two straight needles, with a single thread, through it, so that the points of entry lay in its long axis, and then out through the cheek, knotting the thread over a bolus of lint.

[11] [The large intestine of the ox, prepared so as to leave mostly the peritoneal surface—used to separate the leaves of gold during beating, and also as an adhesive dressing.]

[12] [See n. 5 above.]

15

CHEEK—MELOPLASTY[1]

There are fewer general rules for reconstruction of the cheek, or for closure of holes in it, than for other parts, because the repair must be determined by the nature of the defect. The first attempt to replace a missing cheek was by Gräfe in Germany in 1821.

Case report A man had a large hole in his cheek and the right side of his nose, following attacks of syphilis and gout. His speech was unintelligible unless the hole was covered. Gräfe could not use the skin of the posterior part of the cheek because it was adherent to the underlying tissues. As the skin of the neck was too far away, the choice lay between the forehead and the arm, but the skin of the latter was too thin and delicate. Gräfe made a pattern slightly larger than the defect, and laid it a little to the left side of the forehead to allow the flap to rotate more easily to the right; even the places for the sutures were marked. The flap was raised in the usual way; two vessels near the root of the nose were ligated. The attachment was with eight ligature-rods.[2] The speech was no better immediately after the operation, as the flap was still too soft. The pedicle was divided at 5–6 weeks. Two arteries spurted at the upper edge, and had to be ligated, but the lower edge only oozed; the flap went pale. Several months later, when the patient was completely healed, his appearance was greatly improved, and he could smell again, but his voice, although intelligible, was still affected by the destruction of his palate.[3]

The difficulty of finding material to reconstruct the cheek led Roux to the ingenious method of bringing the flap from a distance.[4]

Case report A woman had lost the left half of the upper lip, the ala, and part of the cheek with the underlying bone. Her tongue prolapsed

---

[1] Also often called genioplasty, although *genion* means the chin. [Surgery of the cheek is sometimes (correctly) called genoplasty.]

[2] [See p. 101, n. 35.]

[3] C. F. von Gräfe, Meloplastik, *J. Chir, Augenheilk.* **2**, 14 (1821).

[4] [Case report by Maisonabe; see p. 155, n. 27.]

through the defect. Seven operations were needed. First, a flap was raised from the lower lip, and attached to the remains of the upper lip, so that this was restored. Two fruitless attempts were made to mobilize the surrounding skin to cover the cheek; similarly with a piece from the upper lip, and one from the palm of the hand, where the weight of the hand tore the flap away. The patient could not tolerate an obturator. Roux then had the idea of freeing the flap from the upper lip, and using it to close the opening by implanting it near the orbit. This succeeded, and the upper lip was then once more reconstructed from the lower lip.

Labat reported Lallemand's technique where there was no rotation of the flap.[5] Recently Nichet described the closure of an old perforation into the mouth.

Case report Several years ago a man aged 25 put a pistol under his chin and shot himself. He was left with a hole one inch in diameter. The anterior margin of this was turned so far inwards that his beard scratched his tongue. His tongue was fixed by scar-tissue, and his speech and swallowing were affected. Nichet raised a flap from the anterior margin (based towards the chin), excised the margins of the defect, and attached the flap with seven sutures and sticking-plaster. It was healed in 21 days, but his speech was no better.[6]

Recently Dieffenbach has closed huge holes in the cheeks, partly by mobilizing all the neighbouring tissues, and partly by true transplantation. These cases are to be described in the fifth section of his book.[7]

---

[5] Labat, *De la rhinoplastie*, p.332.

[6] J. P. Nichet, Coup de feu à la face, perforation du plancher de la bouche, autoplastie, guérison, *Gaz. Méd.* p. 454 (1836).

[7] Dieffenbach, *Erfahrungen*, Vol. 5 (1838) [unpublished].

16

LACRIMAL FISTULA

The difficulty of closing a lacrimal fistula is shown by the large number of operations that have been recommended. Although it is easy to introduce a small tube or other instrument to enlarge the duct, the effect does not last, and the opening into the sac remains. In some cases this can be healed by caustics, scarification, and general measures for any underlying disease, but in others the margins become scarred over, and the fistula is re-established. After simple approximation and suture, the skin does not heal. Dieffenbach therefore tried transplantation.

Case report A woman had had the duct satisfactorily dilated six years before, but the fistula remained. Tears flowed continuously from an opening the size of a lentil. The duct had closed again, and the surrounding skin was red and indurated. Dieffenbach passed a blunt sound through the duct, and put in a lead wire, bringing its lower end out through the nostril. Six weeks later he removed the wire, and raised a bipedicled flap a quarter of an inch broad and one-third of an inch long on the side of the nose. The lower pedicle was broader, and provided the main nourishment for the flap; the upper pedicle was simply to keep the flap stretched out. The posterior margin was attached to the back of the fistula with four fine insect-pins. The gaping wound on the side of the nose was left open to avoid all tension. Cold compresses were applied. The flow of tears stopped, even from the nasal side of the flap, which Dieffenbach had deliberately left attached by a small strip of subcutaneous tissue. There was considerable swelling and redness spreading to the upper eyelid, and erysipelas developed. This took three weeks to resolve, by which time the suppurating wound on the side of the nose had healed. The fistula did not recur.[1]

Dieffenbach has recently used this method successfully in several more cases.

[1] Dieffenbach, *Erfahrungen*, Vol. 2, p. 121 (1830).

17

FILLING THE ORBIT AFTER REMOVAL OF THE EYE

Dieffenbach advised the following operation to improve the appearance of the sunken eyelids after complete removal of the eye, where an artificial eye cannot be worn, as it can with partial destruction of the eye:

The outer commissure is split, and the skin is undermined so that the eyelids can be retracted. A flap is raised at the junction of the temple and the cheek, at least one and a half inches in diameter. It is laid in the orbit, and fixed to the eyelids with 5–6 interrupted sutures, leaving one end of each of these long. Then the lids are drawn together over the flap, and held with sticking-plaster. The wound in the temple is easily closed. The sutures can be removed by pulling on the long ends without the need to separate the lids widely again. Later the pedicle is excised, and this wound is sutured.[1]

---

[1] Dieffenbach, *Erfahrungen*, Vol. 2, p. 133 (1830).

18

SOFT PALATE—STAPHYLOPLASTY[1]

I shall not be dealing here with staphylorrhaphy, because suture of the soft palate is no more a plastic operation than repair of a hare-lip. Besides, Schwerdt gives a comprehensive survey of the subject.[2] It may be objected that I have included, especially under cheiloplasty, operations that also only consist in advancement of tissue for the repair of defects. I can only apologize that it would have taken too much space to describe this important operation in the detail that it deserves, and I shall limit myself to the description of what has been attempted in the true staphyloplasty or palatoplasty.

The difficulty of repair of a cleft of the soft palate[3] raises no great hopes of successful repair of complete loss of the soft palate. But Dieffenbach was bold enough to try:

Case report A girl, whose sunken nose Dieffenbach had previously built up, had no soft palate, except for a band of scar from the left tonsil to the hard palate; there was also a defect in the posterior part of the hard palate. Dieffenbach made an incision, with a scalpel curved on the flat, on the inner side of the right cheek from the end of the hard palate to the tonsil. He then raised a flap on the inside of the left cheek, and freshened the posterior margin of the hard palate, boring two holes through its right side. The flap was attached to this by passing lead wires from front to back through the bone, bringing the ends out of the mouth, threading them on palate needles, and passing them from behind forwards through the flap. Two more wires were inserted to join the flap to the incision in the right cheek. As the flap was under considerable tension, and there was still a gap of one-third of the width of the palate, Dieffenbach lengthened the flap by an incision in the

---

[1] [Zeis used the terms 'staphyloplasty' and 'palatoplasty' for the repair of acquired defects of the palate—usually syphilitic. The repair of complete congenital clefts ('uranoplasty') did not become possible until the work of Langenbeck and others in the 1860s.]

[2] F. R, T. Schwerdt, *Die Gaumennaht*, Berlin, (1829).

[3] [The first successful repair of a cleft of the soft palate was by von Gräfe in Berlin (1816), followed by Roux in Paris (1819).]

cheek. By pulling on the wires, and enlarging this relieving incision, the flap reached the right side. One fine wire suture was put between the hard palate and the flap. The defect was then completely closed. The posterior border of the flap was so close to the tongue that there was hope that she might develop clear speech.

She was forbidden to talk, and allowed only beef-tea and ice-cream, with frequent cold syringing to clear the mucus. All went well at first, but the wound began to gape on the fourth day. On the sixth day the flap gave way, retracting to the left side, leaving only a small attachment that was of little benefit to her.[4]

Schwerdt advises that the incision should be made (with a long scalpel angled on the flat) just behind the last molar tooth, raising a flap from the cheek, and attaching it to the half of the hard palate on the same side. If this unites, the flap is divided, and attached to the other half of the palate. He thinks that, in this way, the flap will heal better than if it is brought directly to the opposite side, when there would be more tension.[5]

For greater surety, Dieffenbach advises that the sutures should be left to become calloused in the wound edges, and only then should repair be carried out.

[4] Dieffenbach, *Erfahrungen*, Vol. 1, p. 49 (1829).
[5] op. cit, p. 47.

19

EAR—OTOPLASTY

Tagliacozzi's chapter on reconstruction of the ear is of particular interest because he took the skin from behind the ear, and not from the arm, and this might be regarded as an example of the Indian method. He described the advantages of using local skin, and it seems therefore that, if he had known of the Indian method of rhinoplasty, he might have preferred it to his own much more laborious method.[1]

Loss of the ear is usually due to a wound, or sometimes a burn. Diseases that destroy the nose or the lips do not affect the ear, so that it is much less commonly deformed. The loss of a small part of the ear can easily be hidden by the hair, and, even when there is not enough for this, a deformity of the ear is not as unsightly as in the nose or lips. Since defects are rare, and we hardly ever cut off an ear as a punishment, there is much less opportunity to restore ears than noses and other parts. The external ear undoubtedly serves to collect sound-waves, so that if it is missing the hearing will suffer. But even if it is not just a question of vanity, and there is real need for otoplasty, there is still the problem that, at least in the present state of the art, although small defects can be repaired, it is very difficult to make a complete ear out of skin. Painted wood or metal is no replacement for a nose, but an ear made of tin, to the pattern of a normal ear and appropriately coloured, outdoes plastic surgery. The obstacles to the solution of this problem lie in the contraction of the skin, and the impossibility of giving cartilaginous support to the reconstruction.

It is less trouble to take the skin from behind the ear than from the arm, and quicker, because the flap can be attached as soon as it has been raised. Tagliacozzi adopted this technique because of the small size of the flap required. He warned strongly of the danger of damaging a large artery behind the ear, although now we do not share his anxiety. He raised the flap in the hairless skin behind the ear. The size of the defect was marked on the skin, but the incision was made a little wider

---

[1] 'For in this way we gain a considerable advantage, in that the transplant, as soon as it recovers from its injuries, acquires an exceptional strength, suckled, as it were, by two udders. Thus it cannot shrink and disappoint the hopes for the operation.' Tagliacozzi, *de curtorum*, Vol. 2, Chapter 20.

to allow for contraction. The flap was undermined down to the periosteum, which had to be preserved. Large arteries were compressed and dressed with tinder.[2] While an assistant took care of this, the surgeon freshened the defect without damaging the cartilage. Then the flap was sutured accurately into place. Great care was needed with the dressings, and a small bolus was placed behind the ear to ensure that the flap was held in place. The sutures were dusted with powder to prevent suppuration. Tagliacozzi gave no instructions for dividing the flap, and, indeed, he said that procedures to improve its shape, as with a rhinoplasty, were not necessary.

I do not know of anyone in recent times, except Dieffenbach, who has attempted to reconstruct an ear. The difficulty is to reproduce the folds and hollows of the normal pinna. A flap will always contract, and it cannot be kept stretched to look like a free-standing ear. It is different when only part of the ear is missing, particularly the lobule which lends itself to replacement by a flap of skin. For this, Dieffenbach makes an incision over the mastoid process, undermines it a little, and attaches it to the freshened defect with insect-pins. When this has healed, he raises as large a piece of skin-off the mastoid as possible, dresses the wound, and covers the raw surface of the now greatly enlarged lobule with ointment. By contraction and spontaneous rounding-off it will reach a shape that can hardly be distinguished from normal. He has also repaired the upper part of the ear in the same way.

Case report A man had had a piece of the top of his ear cut off, half an inch in height and one and a half inches broad. The scarred margin of the defect was excised, and a two-inch incision in the scalp was made parallel to the defect. By incisions one-third of an inch long at either end this was turned into a broad rectangular flap, which was sutured to the ear, with an oily dressing underneath to stop it readhering to its bed. It healed well, and three weeks later Dieffenbach lifted a crescentic piece of skin from the scalp, which was one-third larger than the defect. The flap went pale at first, but quickly recovered; its posterior surface then gradually scarred over. One week after the operation the patient could feel the prick of a needle, and the flap had become the same colour of the rest of the ear.

---

[2] [Amadou, German tinder—prepared from the corkwood fungus, and used as a match and a styptic.]

Since then Dieffenbach has reconstructed several lobules by the 'displacement' method,[3] especially in cases of burns or scrofula where the lower part of the ear has fused with the cheek.

[3] See p. 96, n. 28.

20

TRACHEAL FISTULA—BRONCHOPLASTY

'Bronchoplasty' is the name given by Velpeau, and other French authors, to the closure of a chronic fistula in the trachea. Since attempts to close such fistulae by freshening the edges and suturing nearly always fail, he developed a method of inserting a folded flap into the defect.

Case-report Velpeau's patient was a young man who had cut his throat, but had been revived. The wound had been sutured, but he was left with a hole, between the hyoid and the larynx, big enough to put a finger in. He was ashamed of what he had done, and, when he came under Dupuytren's care at the Hôtel Dieu, he made out that a surgeon had opened his trachea because a potato got stuck in it. Bennati[1] used him for his experiments on the voice, and then Dupuytren tried unsuccessfully to close the opening by excising the edges and putting in twisted sutures. The patient kept the hole filled with lint, but secretions poured out if he did not keep his head bent forwards. He could only speak in a hoarse voice, but even this disappeared if he lifted his chin off his chest. Velpeau wished to help such a young patient, but felt that neither caustics nor the hare-lip operation (paring and advancing the edges, with relieving incisions) would answer the purpose. He recognized that simple skin cover, without underlying tissue, would not prevent the escape of mucus, and he had the idea of putting in a living bung. On 11 February 1832 he raised a flap over the larynx, one inch wide and one and two-thirds inches long, and turned it up, leaving it with a pedicle only one-third of an inch wide. Then he folded it with the skin surfaces together, and laid this cylinder in the freshened fistula, transfixing it with two long needles, and wrapping these round with

[1] [Francesco Bennati (1798–1834), physician to the Opera in Paris, devoted his life to the study of the physiology and pathology of the human voice.]

thread. It healed almost completely, and the patient's voice returned to normal. A small opening that remained was cauterized.[2]

There is no evidence that Velpeau made up this account, but it seems incredible that such a folded flap would heal by first intention.

[2] A. L. M. Velpeau, Fistule laryngienne traitée avec succèss, au moyen d'une opération nouvelle, *Gaz. Hôp, Paris* p. 209 (1832).

21

TRANSPLANTATION OF SKIN TO PREVENT RECURRENCE OF CANCER

Martinet de la Creuse has recently stated that recurrence of cancer after excision can be prevented by covering the area with a skin flap, instead of letting it heal by granulation.[1] If this is true (which I doubt), it would be one of the greatest advances in surgery in recent times. But it can only be established by impartial observation and long experience. Surgeons have always known the value of preserving as much healthy skin as possible to cover a wound—thus, extirpation of the breast is preferable to amputation. This is not done to prevent recurrence, but to shorten the time of healing. It is also recognized that the scirrhous nodules, which are the early signs of recurrence, occur in hard broad scars, so that it is important to ensure a soft narrow scar. Although it has not yet been proved that cancer recurs most commonly when a large area of skin has been removed, Martinet had the idea of healing the wound as quickly as possible by covering it with a flap. He based this on four cases. The account given here is taken from Blandin,[2] because no details have yet appeared in the German journals.

Case 1 The first patient had a mushroom-like growth on the left ala for six years. It had started as a little wart, and then became cracked and crusted, with pain and discharge. Martinet excised it, leaving the cartilage. Nine days later a new growth had formed, larger and more painful than the first. This was excised, and cauterized with arsenic which caused a severe general reaction; the scab had to be removed with a scalpel. After several months it was still unhealed and discharging. Martinet therefore covered the area with a flap from the cheek, attaching it with two sutures. On the eighteenth day it was soundly

[1] Martinet de la Creuse, Mémoire sur un nouveau procédé opératoire à prévenir la récidive du cancer, *Gaz. Méd.* p. 657 (1834).

[2] Blandin, *Autoplastie*, p. 226.

healed, and the pedicle was divided. Six years later there was no recurrence.

Case 2 A woman aged 44, who had no children but who had menstruated regularly up to the age of 40, had had a scirrhous tumour of the right breast for two years. As she had been treated by stimulating remedies the tumour had started to fungate. There were three large glands in the axilla. On 30 March 1830 Martinet excised the tumour and the glands in the usual way, but it recurred five months later. The recurrence was excised with a two-inch margin, exposing the ribs and their cartilages; suspicious areas were cauterized with a red-hot iron. The scab separated on the sixth day, and Martinet covered the defect with a lateral flap on a one-inch pedicle. The patient died two and a half years later of another disease, without recurrence of the cancer.

Case 3 A woman aged 29 had had an injury to the left breast. Three years later, when she came under Martinet's care, she had a hard tumour in the breast, the size of an egg. This was adherent to the skin, but mobile on the deeper tissues; there were no glands. Martinet excised the tumour through a curved incision under the breast, and packed the wound with lint. It healed by granulation, but the skin that had covered the tumour, and had been preserved, began to ulcerate. At a second operation all the diseased tissue was removed. When the wound had granulated, a suspicious area in the centre was treated with caustic potash. After the scab had separated a few days later, Martinet covered the area with a lateral flap. Three years later there was no recurrence.

Case 4 A servant aged 40 had had a hard knotty tumour in the left cheek for three years, which was attached to the skin, and tender on pressure. His appearance was so awful that he could no longer find employment. Martinet excised the tumour, including the mucous membrane of the cheek which was involved. The operation was made more difficult by extensions of the tumour to the pterygoid muscles and the transverse process of the third cervical vertebra. The excision left a large hole, with the tongue protruding through it. The wound was closed with a quilled suture, with the help of relieving incisions. Many arteries had to be ligated, but the blood-loss was relatively slight. The excised tumour was hard, with soft porridge-like areas. Several hours after the operation there was a severe haemorrhage. A new bandage was applied, with a thin lead plate between the jaw and the cheek for counter-pressure. Healing was very slow, and after two months there was extensive recurrence inside the mouth, and the wound broke down. Martinet excised and destroyed all the diseased tissue, partly with a knife and partly with a red-hot iron. When the scab had separated, he transferred a flap from the shaved skin of the back of the head, with its pedicle on the mastoid process. The patient felt reasonably well after this, and there was no cerebral disturbance. When all the swelling had settled, small unhealed areas were freshened and closed with twisted sutures. For some months there was a salivary fistula, but this gradually closed. The patient was left with a linear scar which he could cover with his transplanted beard. The defect in the scalp healed in the usual way, leaving a one-inch scar. After three years there has been no recurrence.

It can be seen that Martinet was not strictly accurate in his diagnosis of cancer. Only the second and third cases had genuine cancer of the breast. His first case was an ulcer resulting from a doubtful warty growth, and the fourth case sounds more like tuberculosis than cancer. Blandin gives these case reports, and adds one of his own in which recurrence of cancer of the nose in a man aged 62 was prevented by a flap.[3] There are several others in the literature that could certainly be used to support Martinet, such as von Ammon's blepharoplasty,[4] but there are just as many to contradict him. Martinet applies the flap some time after the excision, when granulations are already forming; but Blandin advises its immediate application. Martinet attributes the success of his method to the fact that it relieves the tension on the tissues round the wound. Blandin thinks that the flap, by drawing its nourishment from the underlying tissues, will thereby reduce their overactivity. These explanations are not entirely satisfactory. If the facts are proven, I think it is more likely to be that the wound is kept from contact with the air while it is granulating, and that a hard scar, which is commonly the site of recurrence, is avoided. Whether Martinet's idea is true or not, it should be tested further. Even if transplantation only sometimes prevents recurrence, we would all be glad to have any means of limiting this terrible disease.

Reconstruction after cancer of the lip, nose, and other organs is always carried out, whenever it is possible, for other reasons. But Martinet's views lead to the conclusion that a flap should now be used in all cases of cancer of the breast. This could easily be done, without

[3] Blandin, *Autoplastie*, p. 266.

[4] [See pp. 139–40.]

the operation becoming much more traumatic, by making the incisions as an equilateral triangle instead of an oval. A flap could then be transposed, without rotation and without crossing intact skin. Even if the skin over the tumour was healthy, any raw area would be moved to the side, and the flap would prevent suppuration and scarring at the original site of the tumour. As in all plastic operations, the incisions would have to be at right angles through the skin (which is not always done in extirpative operations), so that closure could be made with twisted sutures in the expectation that there would be primary healing. Such an operation would be as easy as Dieffenbach's blepharoplasty or cheiloplasty. The routine treatment after amputation of the breast would have to be altered, as cold compresses must be used to ensure the healing of the flap. Primary healing is not as easy to achieve over a large surface as in a simple incision, but it would not matter if some places suppurated, for syringing and a light pressure dressing would bring about healing.[5]

[5] [Several surgeons followed Martinet's precepts, but it was soon found that the technique did not prevent recurrence, although the advantages of using skin flaps to promote rapid healing were recognized.]

22

FORESKIN—POSTHIOPLASTY[1]

To avoid persecution in the time of the Roman Emperors, Jews are said to have had their foreskins reconstructed. Celsus describes two methods, one for congenital loss, and one for acquired.[2] The naturally short foreskin is treated by pulling the skin forwards until it covers the glans, and holding it there with a ligature. An incision is then made round the penis near the base, denuding the shaft, with care to avoid injuring the urethra. This extensive defect is dressed and allowed to heal by granulation. The ligature must be left until healing is complete, with only a small opening for the urine. If the foreskin has been completely removed by circumcision, a circular incision is made near the glans. The skin is freed from the penis, pulled forwards, and covered with cold compresses to reduce inflammation. The patient must keep to a strict diet. When the inflammation has subsided, the wound is dressed from the base towards the glans to pull the skin over the tip.

Tagliacozzi does not mention this subject, but Jessenius von Jessen describes an operation to lengthen a short foreskin by retracting it and making a circular incision in its lining, taking care to avoid the vessels running between the two layers. A dressing is put between the glans and the foreskin to prevent readhesion, and the skin is pulled down until it covers the glans. A catheter is inserted, and the dressing is renewed until healing is complete.[3] This operation was carried out on Jews who wished to be converted, and to have a new foreskin, so that they were called *recutiti*.[4] Petit has attempted to replace a missing foreskin by incising the skin of the shaft and pulling it forwards, but it contracted and bunched up round the glans.[5]

I do not know whether complete absence of the foreskin can ever be congenital. In hypospadias it is common for the frenulum to be miss-

---

[1] *Posthion*—foreskin.

[2] Celsus, *de medicina*, Book **7,** Chapter 25.

[3] J. von Jessen, *Institutiones chirurgicae*, Vol. 4, Wittenberg ch. 4, p. 104[a] (1601).

[4] Some of the older authors use this term for those who have been circumcised, but others (and this is more correct) use it for those who have had their foreskins reconstructed.

[5] J. L. Petit, *Oeuvres complètes (bibliothèque chirurgicale)*, Vol. 2, Limoges, p. 711 (1837).

ing, with a fold of skin representing the foreskin on the dorsum of the glans. The urethra, particularly if it reaches the glans, can be brought forwards and narrowed by unrolling this fold, pulling it round, and attaching it to the under-surface of the penis where the frenulum should be.

The Jews, and many others where the glans is denuded, show how a man can get used to being without a foreskin. Mere vanity is therefore not a good enough reason for reconstruction. But various forms of syphilis can destroy the foreskin partially or completely, and its replacement may be worthwhile for those patients who find the exposure of the glans to the air unpleasant. Sometimes the foreskin is not so much destroyed as diseased, and it is not to be expected that reconstruction will then be successful. If the skin is adherent to the glans, operation is indicated because coitus is impossible or very painful.

The usual operations for phimosis are not suitable for the complete adhesion of the foreskin to the glans, which is often the result of chronic gonorrhoea, and makes erection painful. In one such case Dieffenbach separated the adhesion with scissors, splitting the foreskin until the whole glans and corona were free. Oily dressings were used, but the adhesion recurred. Dieffenbach then had to remove the whole foreskin.[6] In another case there was more of a reconstruction, so that it could properly be called a posthioplasty.[7]

Case reports In a man whose foreskin was fused to the glans, Dieffenbach separated them, and removed all the diseased skin so that the glans was completely denuded, with a raw surface at the corona. He then made a circular incision two-thirds of an inch behind the corona, turned the skin in, and shifted it up to the corona, where it was held in position with dressings. It healed in two weeks, and the patient was delighted to be freed from a disability that had upset him mentally more than physically.

Encouraged by this success, Dieffenbach treated a 26-year-old schoolmaster with a thickened adherent foreskin from long-standing gonorrhoea. The young man was driven to operation by his anxiety that he could not cohabit fully. The outer layer of the foreskin, which was unusually long, was incised and turned back. The diseased adherent inner layer (as thick as cardboard) was removed, and the outer layer was turned in at the corona, and held with dressings. There

---

[6] Dieffenbach, *Erfahrungen,* Vol. 1, p. 57 (1829).

[7] Ibid. p. 59.

was considerable inflammation, and the raw surface of the glans suppurated. To protect the inner layer of the new foreskin the patient was instructed to irrigate it hourly with tepid lead lotion and infusion of elder. After three weeks everything had healed. When Dieffenbach saw the young man some time later, the inner layer of skin had become thin, red, and moist, so that there must have been the normal secretion under the foreskin.[8] Since then, Dieffenbach has often repeated this operation successfully; the same technique has been used by Svitzer in Copenhagen.[9]

[8] Ibid. p. 63.

[9] E. Svitzer, *Beretnig om nogle Forsog til at danne en ny Forhud. Bibliothek for Laeger, Udgivet af Directionen,* Vol. 5, Copenhagen, p. 40 (1831).

23

SCROTUM—OSCHEOPLASTY[1]

Transplantation of skin after excision of a diseased scrotum, or covering testicles denuded for any other reason, is an important plastic operation to ensure the preservation of such vital organs. The operation has, up to now, been so rarely performed that the few known cases will be described here, rather than any general principles. The most important case was that of Delpech, in 1820, where the scrotum was enormously enlarged by elephantiasis.[2] The plastic part of the operation consisted of retaining enough healthy skin, after excision of the mass, for three flaps—two to make the scrotum and cover the testicles, and one to cover the penis. The normal skin of the scrotum is very flexible, as seen in every scrotal hernia, so that even in large defects it can be pulled together, and there is no need to bring a flap from a distance. But if there is such loss of tissue that a new scrotum has to be reconstructed, some other method than Delpech's will have to be devised. The last part of his operation, covering the penis with skin, is quite distinct from oscheoplasty, and it needs a new name.

Case-report Authier, a man aged 35 from Perpignan, father of several healthy children, had been a soldier in Portugal when he was only 14 years old. Four years later he became a butcher, and got a gonorrhoea which disappeared after treatment with mercury. At the age of 27 he noticed a small ulcer on his foreskin; this was cauterized, causing severe pain and inflammation. He then had a course of mercurial inunctions, but the ulcer did not heal, and, as he had to ride a lot, the pain and inflammation increased. In two months, swelling spread over the whole foreskin and into the scrotum which became doughy and then hard. The penis disappeared in the swelling, and the testicles could not be felt; there was a sort of navel which was the opening of the urethra. No other part of his body was involved. Seven years after the onset of

---

[1] *oschos*—bag, purse, or pouch.

[2] J. M. Delpech, Observation d'un cas d'intumescence énorme du scrotum, symptome d'éléphantiasis, *Chirurgie clinique*, **2,** 5 (Paris, 1828). [See also: T. Gibson, Delpech: His contributions to plastic surgery and the astonishing case of scrotal elephantiasis, *Br. J. plast, Surg.* **9,** 4 (1956).]

the disease he was sent to Montpellier. The swelling hung down to his calves from a pedicle 18 inches in circumference.

Delpech saw him on 1 August 1820, and operated on 1 September. The patient was laid flat and restrained by assistants. The tumour was held in a table-cloth so that two assistants could raise or lower it as necessary. Three flaps were made: an anterior (*a*), which had five sides and a sixth as its base, and two lateral (*b, b*) [Fig. 40]. The spermatic cords were easily distinguished from the abnormal tissue, and were followed down to the testicles which lay twelve inches from the inguinal rings. The testicles looked healthy, and retained their normal sensation; this part of the operation caused the patient severe pain. The corpora cavernosa were hard to find, but Delpech put his finger in the sinus from which the urine flowed, and followed this to the glans, before freeing the penis with a layer of healthy tissue. He was anxious not to leave any diseased tissue, and he dissected the mass out of the perineum with great care. Many arteries had to be ligated; as there were so many of them the threads were cut close to the knots. The spermatic cords were so long that they had to be laid zigzag. The lateral flaps were brought over the testicles, and their posterior four-fifths were joined with interrupted sutures onc inch apart. The anterior flap was wrapped round the penis, with the middle two sides sutured to each other in the midline; the distal side overlapped the glans as the free border of the prepuce, and the proximal two sides were sutured to the anterior fifth of the lateral flaps [Fig. 41].

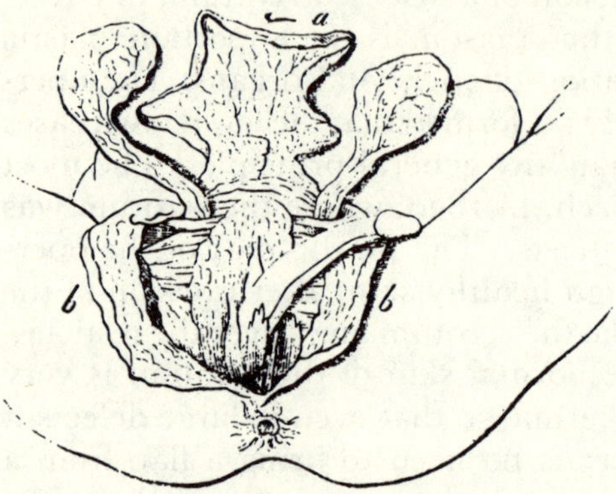

Fig. 40

The operation took 57 minutes. The patient was given 60 drops of laudanum, as Delpech felt that it was important to relieve him of pain as soon as possible. The wound was covered with greasy dressings, padding, and a T-bandage, leaving only the penis exposed. The tumour weighed 54 pounds; about six pounds of fluid were lost during the operation.

His pulse was weak at first, and his limbs cold, but he was conscious. He soon warmed up, and his pulse improved. At first he could not pass water, but this recovered the next day. A small patch of skin on the penis became gangrenous, but the general swelling was moderate. The edges of the wound healed in most places, but in others there was suppuration which lasted longest in the right inguinal region. But it was always laudable, and good granulations developed. In the third week there was induration in the new scrotum; this was poulticed, and an abscess discharged. The ligatures were gradually extruded, and the patient began to walk about. His penis seemed to be normally only two inches long, but it lengthened with erections day by day.

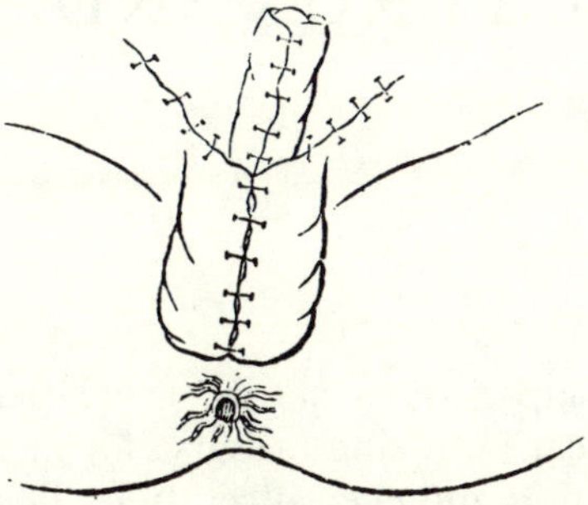

Fig. 41

By the end of November everything had healed, but Delpech kept him in hospital for another two months for observation. He was then discharged because he wanted to get back to his family, but also because he was abusing the increased freedom that he was given, and had taken to the bottle. Unfortunately he died suddenly from an abscess of the liver several weeks after he got home.

Dieffenbach also did an operation that deserves to be included here, although it consisted only of using the abnormally retracted skin of the scrotum to cover a denuded testicle.

Case-report A 30-year-old professor, with recurrent abdominal disease and inflammation of the liver, lost half his scrotum from gangrene. The right testicle was exposed, and it was feared that it might become diseased, so that castration would be necessary. Dieffenbach freed the skin where it had become adherent to the spermatic cord, covered the testicle, and sutured the edges of the scrotum. Although there was severe swelling and suppuration, union occurred in enough places to prevent prolapse of the testicle. It was completely healed in four weeks.[3]

Thus there was no transplantation of the skin from the thigh or the belly in either of these cases. Labat reported a similar case of his own,[4] and two of Clot-Bey, one of which[5] was not much different from Delpech's, but in the other[6] the skin to cover the penis was taken from the original penile skin which, as it is hairless, is more appropriate. Seerig operated exactly as Delpech.[7]

---

[3] Dieffenbach, *Erfahrungen,* Vol. 2, p. 137 (1830).

[4] Labat, *De la rhinoplastie,* p. 336 (1834).

[5] A.-B. Clot-Bey, *Histoire d'une tumeur éléphantiaque du scrotum du poids de 110 livres, extirpée avec succés chez un Arabe*, Marseilles, (1830).

[6] A.-B. Clot-Bey, Observation d'une tumeur éléphantiaque du scrotum de 50 livres, extirpée avec succès', *Gaz. Hôp. Paris* p. 488 (1833).

[7] W. Seerig, Fall von Elephantiasis scroti, *Magazin ges. Heilk.* **47**, 119 (1836).

24

PROLAPSE OF THE UTERUS AND VAGINA

EPISIORRHAPHY[1]

Fricke's technique for long-standing prolapse is to suture the labia together.[2] This relieves the disability of wearing a ring-pessary, for any foreign body in the vagina can cause irritation and even ulceration. The patient, especially if she is working-class, then has to remove the device. The prolapsed parts soon become diseased, making her weak and feverish, and unfit for all work. Partial closure of the labia will control a reducible prolapse, and it is a relatively minor operation.

After the vulva has been shaved, the patient is put in the lithotomy position, but without securing her hands and feet. The labium majus is transfixed two finger-breadths from the anterior commissure and at least one finger-breadth from its edge. This strip is then quickly excised back to one finger-breadth behind the fourchette. Fricke recommends that the strip on each side should be several finger-breadths wide. After twisting the spurting vessels, the wound is closed with 10–12 sutures. A catheter is inserted for the first few days.

The opening that is left at the upper end is adequate for menstrual fluid and vaginal secretions, and even for coitus. If pregnancy results, the adhesion can easily be divided to allow delivery.[3] Union does not always occur, but even a bridge several fingers wide is enough to prevent prolapse. If union fails completely, the operation can easily be repeated. Koch used quilled sutures, with four-inch rolls of sticking-plaster in the loops of the threads.[4]

---

[1] *epision*—the pudendal region.

[2] J. C. G. Fricke, Die Episiorhaphie bei Vorfällen der Mutterscheide und Gebärmutter, *Annalen der chirurgischen Abtheilung des allgemeinen Krankenhauses in Hamburg*, **2**, 142 (1833).

[3] Plath, Geschichte einer Geburt nach gemachter Episiorhaphie, *Z. ges. med.* **2**, 442 (1836).

[4] L. Koch, Ein Beitrag zur Episiorhaphie, *J. Chir, Augenheilk.* **25**, 667 (1837).

ELYTRORRHAPHY[5]

Marshall Hall[6] and Ireland[7] tried to achieve the same result by excising longitudinal strips of mucosa to narrow the vagina. They and Bérard call this 'elytrorrhaphy'. One-and-a-half-inch wide strips are excised from the side-walls of the vagina, from the labia to the cervix. Bleeding is controlled by torsion, and the wounds are sutured. The excisions are made at the sides to avoid injury to the bladder and rectum. Bérard operated on two women, but, in one, the wound failed to unite even when the operation was repeated.[8] Dieffenbach has used the same method in many cases, after he noticed that prolapse did not recur when the vagina had been narrowed by the destruction by gangrene of part of its lining.[9]

COLPODESMORRHAPHY[10]

Bellini used a different technique in a Jewess aged 40 with prolapse involving the rectum. He seated the patient on the edge of a bed, and grasped the swelling with a double hook. Starting at the posterior commissure of the vagina, he passed double-threaded curved needles to raise a large fold of vaginal mucous membrane, keeping one finger in the rectum to avoid injuring it. The result was excellent. A piece of the mucosa sloughed after 10 days, but a scar formed in the vagina, and there was no recurrence.[11]

OPENING UP THE VAGINA

Operations to open up a completely scarred vagina, which are the opposite of those just described, are still too rarely carried out for any general principles to be laid down. Amussat's technique is not enough of a plastic operation to be given in detail here.[12]

---

[5] *elutron*—vagina.

[6] Hall, Marshall, Case of prolapsus uteri cured by a new operation, *Lond. med. Gaz.* **9**, 269 (1832).

[7] Ireland, Case of procidentia uteri successfully treated by operation, *Dubl. J. med. chem. Sci.* **6**, 484 (1835).

[8] A. Bérard, Chute de la matrice, élytrorhaphie, *Gaz. Méd.* 541 (1835).

[9] J. F. Dieffenbach, Ueber Mutterkränze und Radicalcur des Scheiden- und Gebärmuttervorfalles, *Preuss. med. Verztg.* 151 (1836).

[10] *colpos*—vagina.

[11] G. Bellini, Colpodesmorafia, o sia suora operazione per la cura del prolasso della vagina come dell' utero, *Omod. Ann, univ.* **79**, 180 (1836).

[12] J. Z. Amussat, Observation sur une opération de vagin artificiel pratigée avec succès, par un nouveau procédé, suivie de quelques réflexions sur les vices de conformation du vagin, *Gaz. Méd.* 785 (1835). [Amussat bored a passage to the uterus using only his finger.]

25

URETHRAL FISTULA—URETHROPLASTY

The pathology and management of urethral fistula are dealt with in surgical textbooks. Here I shall only consider the applications of plastic surgery, mainly from the work of Dieffenbach.[1] A fistula in the perineum heals relatively easily, if the urine is diverted by a catheter for long enough, because of the thickness of the tissues. It is quite different in the shaft of the penis where the skin is thin, and the flow of urine destroys granulations more quickly than any other fluid. Sometimes the urethra is congenitally split; this has a very poor prognosis. Healing of a fistula depends less on its size than on its proximity to the scrotum. But the nearer the opening is to the scrotum the more the patient wets himself. Semen also comes through a fistula, except when it is very small, and this is depressing for the patient.

Small fistulae run obliquely from behind forwards, and the internal opening is larger than the external. If a small opening cannot be found, the patient is asked to pass water while the glans is compressed—a drop of urine will be seen, or it will mark a piece of linen put over the site. The opening is dilated with a piece of catgut, and then a sound is passed. To get an impression of the internal opening a catheter can be used with a ball of wax on the tip.

It may seem easy to cure a small fistula, but there are many problems. Cauterization with tincture of cantharides can be carried out, with a bougie in the urethra to prevent the caustic running into it. A fine brush is used to paint part of the walls of the fistula. This is repeated three times in 6–8 hours, the bougie is removed, and a catheter is left in the bladder. More caustic is applied after a few days. Dieffenbach has been able to reduce the size of large fistulae in this way, but even if the external opening heals, it breaks down again with a strong stream of urine or after sexual intercourse. He also tried interrupted sutures after cauterization, passing the needle as deeply as possible to include the internal opening, but this always led to severe

---

[1] J. F. Dieffenbach, Ueber die Heilung widernatürlicher Oeffnungen in dem vordern Theile der Harnröhre nach neuen Methoden, *Z. ges. med.* **2**, 1 (1836).

inflammation. It was the same with twisted sutures, and with sutures alone without cauterization. One case in which he made relieving incisions was followed by such severe inflammation that several bleedings were required. He has also given up puncturing the urethra behind the fistula and leaving a catheter in the opening.

Case report A merchant's clerk, with gonorrhoea and chancres, weakened by debauchery, developed generalized syphilis, which was cured by inunctions [of mercury] and Zittmann's decoction.[2] He was left with a large hole in his urethra. Dieffenbach excised the margins in diamond shape (*a*), undermined the edges, and joined them with twisted sutures [Fig. 42]. He then made relieving incisions (*b*, *b*), undermining them so that, when the bridge was lifted, the catheter could be seen in the urethra. In spite of nocturnal erections, union had occurred by the fourth day, as there was no tension on the sutures. Some urine leaked round the catheter, but it was all healed in 15 days.

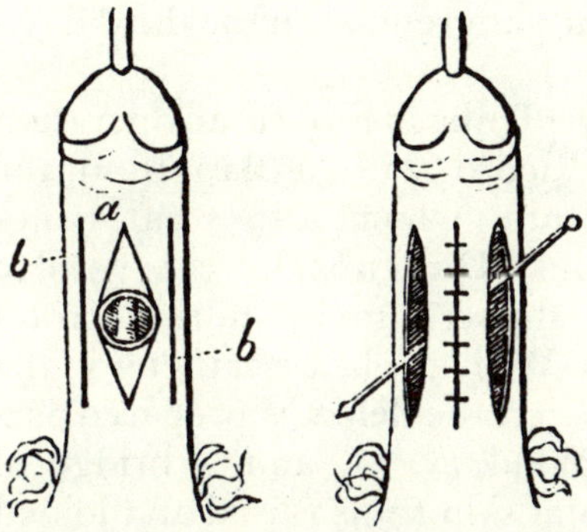

Fig. 42

THE SPLINT SUTURE

Based on the observation that preputial skin does not heal well, but that it will adhere to deeper tissues, Dieffenbach has recommended something similar to the quilled suture, although he has not yet tried this out. The operation will be carried out as above, but the bridge flaps are united by a continuous suture. Two narrow strips of fairly stiff leather, pierced with three holes, are laid along the bridge to hold the flaps together. Needles are passed through the leather and through both flaps, and their ends are turned up. But the tension must not be so great as to kill the skin when it swells. If the penis is very small, so that a single dorsal incision is made, instead of the two lateral incisions, there would be a danger that urine trickling past the catheter could not escape.

TRANSPLANTATION OF SKIN.

Many attempts have been made to transplant skin over a penile fistula. Blandin suggested that the flap should be rolled on itself,[3] as Velpeau

[2] [See p. 61, n, 11.]

[3] Blandin, *Autoplastie*, 180 (1836).

does for the trachea,[4] but he gives no results. Delpech took skin from the inguinal region without success.

Case report A man of twenty-two had wet the bed as a child. Threats and harsh treatment had made him decide one night to tie a string round his penis, but the next morning it had cut in so deeply that the floor of the urethra near the scrotum was destroyed. With a catheter in place, Delpech raised an inguinal flap, and attached its tip to the posterior half of the fistula, but it became gangrenous on the third day.[5]

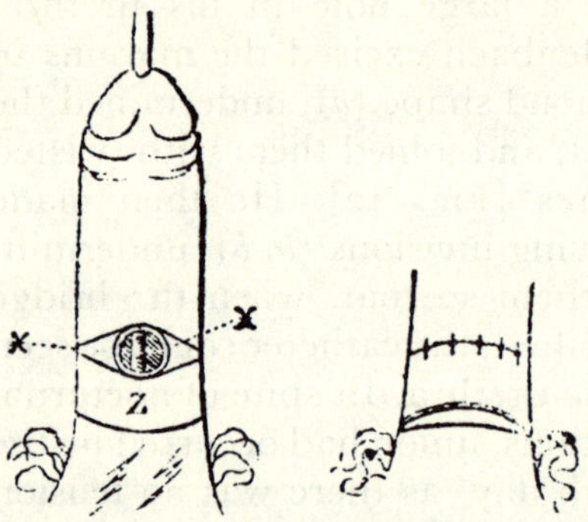

Fig. 43

Dieffenbach reports an operation by Ricord with a flap from the scrotum, which also went gangrenous.[6] Dieffenbach treats fistulae near the scrotum by shifting scrotal skin. With an elastic catheter in the bladder, the defect is prepared as a diamond (*x, x*), and a bridge of scrotal skin (*z*) is raised and joined to the skin of the penis with twisted sutures [Fig. 43]. A two-inch piece of elastic bougie is laid under the flap so that any leaking urine can escape. This method is better than a single-pedicled flap, which tends to contract.

ROTATING THE SKIN OF THE PENIS ON ITS AXIS

There are many ways of shifting penile skin to cover a fistula. For large defects with shortage of skin, Dieffenbach frees the skin round the opening without removing any of it, pulls up a longitudinal fold at the base of the penis, and incises it. The resulting wound must be two-thirds of the circumference of the shaft (*a*) [Fig. 44]. A similar incision is made on the opposite side near the corona (*b*). The skin between these incisions is undermined with sharp scissors. This ring of skin is now twisted so that healthy skin from the dorsum covers the fistula, and the opening in the skin is moved round to the back. The skin is held in position with interrupted sutures and sticking-plaster. Bleeding must

---

[4] [See p. 177, n. 2.]

[5] Delpech, *Chirurg. clinique* **2**, 581 (1828).

[6] Dieffenbach, Ueber die Heilung, p. 27 (1836). [Astley Cooper was the first to use a flap from the scrotum: A. P. Cooper and B. Travers, *Surgical essays* Vol. 2, London, p. 196 (1819).]

be carefully controlled, to ensure that there is no blood-clot between the skin and the shaft. A piece of elastic bougie is laid under the skin as a drain. After the operation a skilled assistant must stay near at hand to cut the plaster if the patient has an erection.

ANTERIOR FISTULAE

Here Dieffenbach uses the outer layer of the foreskin, which is incised around two-thirds of the circumference of the shaft in front of the fistula. A similar incision is made in the skin of the penis behind the fistula, so that the two incisions meet at their ends. The skin around the fistula is excised. An opening for a drain is made in the inner layer of the foreskin where it is attached to the glans. The outer layer of the foreskin is then sutured to the skin of the shaft.

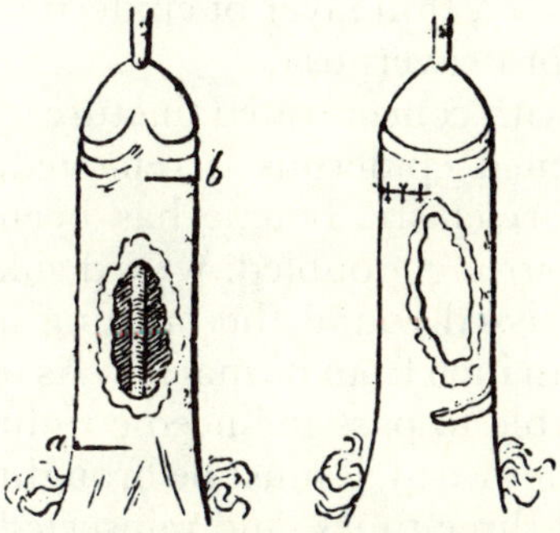

Fig. 44

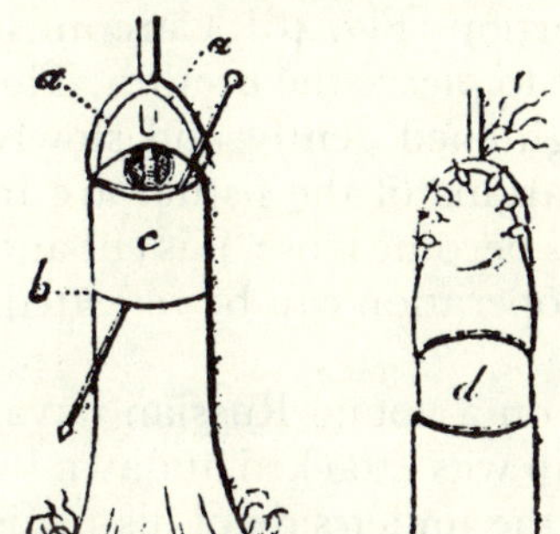

Fig. 45

Closure of large openings immediately behind the glans is one of the hardest operations in surgery. There is nowhere to attach a flap, the margins of the opening are scarred, and a chancre has often destroyed the foreskin before eating into the urethra. It is even more difficult in Jews, for their circumcision removes not only both layers of the prepuce but part of the penile skin as well. In such cases, Dieffenbach bends the glans down to bring the edges together, and joins them with two interrupted sutures; one end of these is cut, and the other is brought out through the urethra on a blunt needle. The skin around the fistula is excised together with the whole undersurface of the glans (*a, a*) [Fig. 45]. The incision *b* is made in the skin of the penis with its ends directed forwards. This bridge, *c*, is undermined, pulled forward over the fistula and sutured. The raw surface, *d*, is dressed with lint. In one of Dieffenbach's cases the repair was destroyed by erections, but another, operated on in Paris, was cured.

THE PURSE-STRING SUTURE

It is clear that many attempts to cure urethral fistulae by transplantation fail, and that healing, when it occurs, is accompanied by violent symptoms which may be life threatening. The indefatigable and ingenious Dieffenbach realized that it was extravasation of urine (even through a needle-hole in the skin) that ruined the operation and caused major complications. He therefore sought a new technique that would not expose the tissues to contact with urine. The purse-string suture is the least traumatic of all surgical operations, and, even if it fails, it cannot make the patient worse off. It is only impracticable when the fistula is immediately behind the glans, or when the surrounding skin is unhealthy or destroyed, so that there is only a thin layer of epidermis adherent to the fibrous sheath of the corpora cavernosa.

The margins of the opening are painted with concentrated tincture of cantharides. The next morning the loosened epidermis is removed. After a short elastic bougie has been inserted, a strong, doubled, waxed silk thread is passed round the opening a quarter of an inch from its margin. As it is not possible to pass the needle right round in one sweep, it must be brought out at least three times, and reinserted in the same hole, until it emerges at the original insertion [Fig. 46]. Care must be taken not to pierce the urethra. The thread is tightened gently and slowly until the margins of the fistula are in contact. After five days, when the thread has become loose, it is cut and removed. If the fistula has not healed, the operation can be repeated.

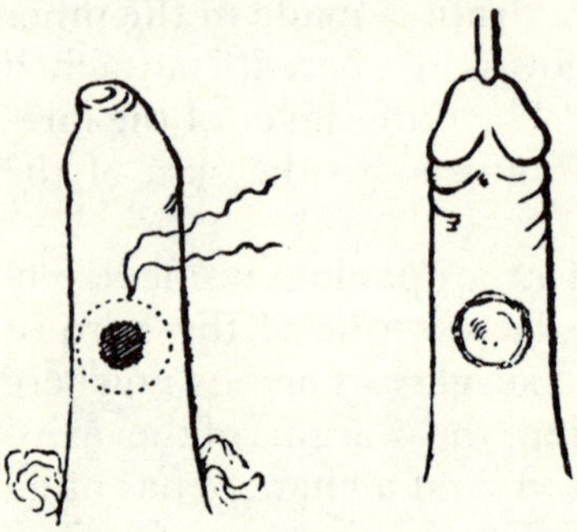

Fig. 46

Case report Dieffenbach used this method on a young Russian naval officer who was asleep on deck when his ship was attacked at dawn by Greek pirates. A bullet tore a piece out of the under side of his penis (which was erect at the time), before penetrating the inguinal region and thigh. When his wounds had healed, he was left with a large fistula. Several years later Dieffenbach operated on him. The purse-string suture caused very little pain or swelling; it loosened and was removed on the seventh day. There was no leakage of urine. Later Dieffenbach noticed a small drop of urine on the scar; the cure was completed by touching with cantharides.

Dieffenbach discovered the purse-string suture by careful observation of natural healing; his operation copies Nature's method of healing other sorts of fistula. The most favourable results can be expected from it in the future.

26

VESICO-VAGINAL FISTULA—CYSTOPLASTY[1] or ELYTROPLASTY[2]

Vesico-vaginal fistula occurs most commonly after difficult childbirth, and poor treatment during this. Sometimes it is due to wounds, catheterization, faulty pessaries, stones, lithotomy, or ulcers. Large fistulae are not always caused by instrumentation, but often by the pressure of the baby's head. A very small fistula cannot be attributed to injury by forceps; it is always in a fold of the mucosa, and Dieffenbach assumes that it arises by the tearing of a mucosal gland when the vagina is stretched, breaking through into the bladder a few days later.

Fistulae are usually near the midline; only in the upper part of the vagina are they sometimes lateral. But whether the fistula is large or small, most of the urine escapes through it. Dieffenbach has described the miserable condition of the patients.[3] There is no relief to be gained from any mechanical device; sponges and containers are only temporary. These fistulae have little natural tendency to heal, and this makes all operations more difficult. Cauterization and simple suture are ineffective, especially in long-standing fistulae, for the flow of urine destroys early union and prevents the formation of granulations. The cure is therefore one of the hardest exercises of our art.

THE PURSE-STRING SUTURE

Dieffenbach tried a purse-string suture in a young Russian woman. She had been so injured at her confinement that her vagina was completely

---

[1] The term 'cystoplasty', like 'bronchoplasty' and 'urethroplasty', implies too much [i.e. that the bladder is being reconstructed]. It would be more correct to use it for the operation that Delpech has suggested for ectopia vesicae (*Chirurgie clinique* **2**, p. 254 (1829)), using a hypogastric flap to make the anterior wall of the bladder. It is doubtful whether this would be so successful that urine would be retained in a bladder without a sphincter, but it would still be a great relief to the patient if the mucosa of the bladder was no longer inflamed by contact with the air.

[2] *elutron*—vagina

[3] J. F. Dieffenbach, Ueber die Heilung der Blasen-Scheiden-Fisteln und Zerreissungen der Blase und Scheide, *Preuss. med. Verztg.* pp. 117, 173 (1836).

occluded. A surgeon, in attempting to open it up, made a hole into her bladder. Dieffenbach first restored the vagina by tents, and then put a purse-string suture round the fistula without freshening or cauterizing the margins. This, and a second attempt, failed. In another case he freshened the margins first, but the patient died on the fourth day of fulminating cystitis. Post-mortem examination showed that the margins were adherent.

SUTURE AFTER EXCISING THE MARGINS

In the next case, a woman aged 28, the fistula was so large that Dieffenbach could not identify it at first, as he put his finger straight into the bladder. He separated the vagina from the bladder, and excised a thin strip round the margins of the fistula to make a broad raw surface for seven interrupted sutures. A catheter was left in the bladder. Four weeks later a small leak in the scar was treated by a purse-string suture; this had to be repeated before she was completely healed.

This is the best method when the fistula is within reach; it is only inferior to the purse-string when the margins are very thin and lax. In contrast to other surgeons, Dieffenbach recommends inserting a large number of interrupted sutures to excite a vigorous inflammatory reaction, to keep the wound edges in close contact, and to prevent urine leaking through.

TRANSPLANTATION

Jobert, as reported by Blandin,[4] was the first to try transplantation, using a flap from the inner surface of the labium majus on a pedicle one-third of an inch wide. The flap was doubled and sutured to itself with its mucosal surfaces together. This fleshy bung was pulled into the fistula by a thread which was passed through the urethra on a catheter, and secured to a T-bandage. A catheter was left in the bladder, and the patient was ordered to stay on her back. Over the next few days she made no complaint except about her position. On the eighth day a strong stream of urine pushed the catheter out. An intern tried to put it back, but found an obstruction at the neck of the bladder. Jobert thought that the 'tampon' had come through the fistula, and was lying at the internal meatus. When everything had healed, the flap was found to be lying as a rounded mass in front of the much reduced fistula. The patient was improved, but not cured. It seems unlikely that such an

[4] Blandin, *Autoplastie*, p. 83.

operation would be completely successful when the flap was not sutured into place.

Later, Jobert[5] did the operation differently (apparently on the same woman), taking the flap from the crease between the thigh and the buttock, with its base above. After 10 days the patient could pass urine normally. At four weeks the flap was divided one inch from its base. After several months the patient was well, and it was hoped that she was completely cured, but it would have been better if Jobert had waited longer before publishing the case, until he was sure of this. In another case of Jobert's, the flap from the labium majus grew hair which caused very unpleasant irritation in the vagina, and interfered with coitus.

DIEFFENBACH'S TECHNIQUE

If the fistula is of medium size, with a fold of the bladder lying near the opening, Dieffenbach paints the margins frequently with cantharides, and pulls the mucosa into the opening with a fine hook. If it adheres, he touches it with silver nitrate to turn it into a tough membrane.

When a large part of the vault of the vagina has been destroyed, so that there is no possibility of bringing the edges together with sutures, he excises a narrow strip of the margin of the fistula, and separates the bladder from the vagina. Then he puts two lead wires (on which needle points have been screwed, as he uses for the palate) through the vaginal edges, not picking up the bladder, and gradually pulls them tight. If there is much tension he makes lateral flaps, by incisions in the postero-lateral walls of the vagina, with his left index finger in the rectum. The width of this isolated strip must be at least one-quarter of the width of the vagina. If the edges can now be brought together easily by pulling on the wires, he closes the wound with interrupted sutures on a curved needle, using a needle-holder for the posterior sutures if they are difficult by hand. The wires are then pulled tight and cut short.

Recently he has operated on many cases of fistula, using a purse-string suture more often than any other method. Apart from this, there was one case in which he was able to unroll, and reattach, a torn flap of vaginal mucosa, which had contracted after 18 years into a small button behind the fistula.

---

[5] A.-J. Jobert, Sur les fistules vesico-vaginales, *Gaz. Méd*, p. 145 (1836).

27

ARTIFICIAL ANUS[1]

The general surgical measures for the cure of an artificial anus[2] will be omitted. The time for plastic surgery is when the obstruction in the gut has been relieved, but the opening has still not closed. Transplanting a skin flap is more effective than simple suture after freshening the edges.

Dieffenbach has been much concerned with this problem, sometimes transplanting skin,[3] and sometimes using a purse-string suture, but his full results have not yet been published.[4] Collier treated a patient whose hernia had been mistaken for an abscess, and opened by an ignorant surgeon. All attempts by this surgeon to close the artificial (or rather the un-artificial) anus had failed. Collier freshened the edges, and transplanted a piece of skin, fixing it with four sutures. It healed completely.[5]

[1] Labat, quite incorrectly, calls the plastic closure of an artificial anus 'proctoplasty'.

[2] [Gastric and intestinal fistulae—the commonest cause of a fistula in the inguinal region was a neglected hernia.]

[3] [Using single and bipedicled flaps.]

[4] J. F. Dieffenbach, Heilung eines schwierigen Falles von künstlichem After durch einen Lanzenstich hervorgebracht, nach einer neuen Methode, *Caspers Wschr.* p. 265 (1834).

[5] Collier, Heilung eines künstlichen Afters durch Hautüberpflanzung, *J. Chir, Augenheilk.* **2,** 655 (1821).

28

HERNIA

Surgeons have always striven to achieve the radical cure of hernias. Ligature of the neck of the sac (the 'Royal Suture')[1], cauterization, caustics, and castration have all been used without certainty of success, or, if they sometimes succeed, the price for cure is too high and the operation is too dangerous.

TRANSPLANTATION OF LOCAL SKIN

Dzondi raised a flap, denuded it of epidermis as far as was necessary, and set it into the hernial ring, which had been scarified.[2] Finck[3] reported a similar operation by Jameson in Baltimore:

A woman had had a herniotomy for a strangulated femoral hernia, which had recurred. A lancet-shaped flap of the skin of the thigh, two inches long and three-quarters of an inch wide, based above, was 'forced into the femoral aperture', and the skin edges were sutured over it, with complete cure.[4]

The success of these two cases means that this technique should be repeated. It must be remembered, as a general principle, that a flap which is to be completely buried in the tissues must have its epidermis removed. There is still the question whether this procedure should immediately follow the operation for a strangulated hernia, or whether it should be done later. When patients recognize the danger that they were in, they can be expected to consent to a further operation that gives them hope of complete cure. It is more difficult to persuade a patient whose hernia has never incarcerated.

TRANSPLANTATION OF OMENTUM

The operation that Blandin calls '*autoplastie herniaire*' is quite different. He inserts omentum in the hernial orifice.[5] There is not much that the

[1] [A ligature placed round the neck of the sac to excite an inflammatory reaction.]

[2] C. H. Dzondi, *Kurze Geschichte des klinischen Institutes,* Halle, p. 117 (1818).

[3] Ph. Finck, *Ueber radicale Heilung reponibler Brüche,* Freiburg, p. 25 (1837).

[4] [G. Jameson, On the permanent cure of femoral hernia, *Lancet,* **2,** 142 (1829-30).]

[5] Blandin, *Autoplastie,* p. 91.

surgeon can do to ensure that this operation is a success—which happens sometimes by chance.

INSERTION OF GOLD-BEATER'S SKIN[6]

Belmas, after many experiments on dogs, concluded that a little bladder of gold-beater's skin, filled with air and inserted into a serous cavity, causes irritation and a profuse exudate, which turns into a dense mass of fibrous tissue. This will close a hernial orifice, and induce adhesions to the surrounding tissues; after a certain time the bladder itself is absorbed. Later, however, Belmas abandoned this technique as too traumatic, and inserted only a very narrow strip of the material into an opening made in the sac. The strip was stuck on to a thin cylinder of dried gelatine which was soon absorbed.[7] But the absorption of the gold-beater's skin takes several months, and it only excites an adhesive inflammation in the area with which it is in contact; this is in contrast to a ligature round the neck of the sac, which excites a suppurative inflammation.

INVAGINATION OF THE SCROTUM

Gerdy has attempted the radical cure of reducible inguinal hernia in men by filling the hernial orifice and the canal with a living bung of part of the scrotum, to excite an adhesive inflammation.

The surgeon stands between the patient's legs, which are held by assistants, and carries out taxis. With his left index-finger he pushes the scrotal skin as high as possible into the canal. Then he passes a [threaded] needle, which has an eye just behind the tip, along the palmar surface of his finger. The needle pierces the anterior wall of the canal until its eye comes through the skin. A little care is needed to avoid injuring the spermatic cord, the epigastric artery, and the hernial sac. One end of the thread is freed, and the needle is pulled back and reinserted to bring the other end out on the skin a little way away from the first. The ends are tied over a small rod, like a quilled suture. If the canal is very wide, two or three such sutures are inserted; usually only one is needed. The invaginated scrotal skin is now cauterized with

---

6 [See p. 166, n. 11.]

7 D.-G. Belmas, *Recherches sur un moyen de déterminer des inflammations adhésives dans les cavités séreuses,* Paris (1829) [and see: On the development of adhesions of serous membranes, and their application to several surgical diseases, *Br. for. med. Rev,* **6,** 232 (1838).]

caustic ammonia. The patient is put back to bed with his scrotum supported, and his bowels are confined while the suture is in place. Local inflammation soon sets in, and the wound starts to suppurate on the third day. Pus is discharged along the suture, which acts as a drain. The suture can now be removed, unless the patient has a cough, when it should be left until the fourth or fifth day. If the local reaction is severe, Gerdy uses potato poultices or leeches, with venesection for any general reaction. There is a risk of chest infection if cooling to prevent peritonitis is carried out too vigorously. But a certain degree of inflammation is necessary for a successful cure, and for the scrotal skin to become adherent. Suppuration usually stops 15–20 days after the operation. The patient must lie on his back for a month, and keep to a light diet. He should then wear a truss for several months. The swelling gradually disappears, leaving only an inconspicuous scar, with the scrotum shortened on that side.

At first Gerdy used sutures to join the invaginated skin, but he found that the cauterization was enough to close off this opening. He has done this operation 30 times, with good results.[8] As far as I know, it has not yet been used in Germany, but it seems to deserve more attention than has been paid to it up to now.

[8] Finck, op. cit. p. 33 [and see: On the radical cure of hernia, *Br. for. med. Rev.* **6,** 341 (1838).

29

TENOTOMY, CLUB-FOOT, WRYNECK

Shortening of tendons gives rise to many pathological conditions. Sometimes deformities are due to this alone, and sometimes it is only part of the problem. Tenotomy is a safe method of treatment. It may not be the complete cure, but it facilitates the mechanical methods which restore parts to normal. Earlier surgeons divided the tendon of the sterno-mastoid, but the operation was then forgotten, and it was only revived towards the end of the previous [eighteenth] century. The literature on this has been reviewed by von Ammon.[1] A number of surgeons then carried out various tenotomies. Michaelis claimed better results from partial than from complete division of the tendons in eight cases.[2] But none of these surgeons gave the subject the attention that it deserved, until it was taken up by Delpech, in 1816, who divided the Achilles tendon for a club-foot, although he was advised against this as being too risky. It seems that he did not know of the work of his predecessors, and he did not often repeat the operation, but he was the first to lay down rules for it.[3]

Since then the operation has been more generally taken up, first in Germany and then in France. Surgeons were held back from it, not because they doubted the value of dividing the tendon in club-foot, but by the fear of complications, such as trismus and tetanus, sloughing of the tendon, or the possibility that the ends would not unite, This last was due to ignorance of the physiology of the healing of divided tendons, which has now been elucidated by von Ammon in experiments on horses and rabbits.[4] He showed that the gap between the cut ends fills first with blood clot. Granulations then grow out of the ends, and the clot becomes more and more organized, while the granulations

---

[1] F. A. von Ammon, *Commentatio chirurgica de physiologia tenotomiae experimentis illustrata*, Dresden (1837).

[2] H. S. Michaelis, Ueber die Schwächung der Sehnen durch Einschneidung, *J. prakt. Arzneik. Wundarzneik.* **23,** 1 (1811).

[3] J. M. Delpech, *Chirurgie clinique de Montpellier,* **1,** 147 (Paris, 1828).

[4] Von Ammon, op. cit.

elongate until they meet. This new connective tissue gradually becomes less vascular, and the whole mass is converted into tendinous fibres, so that there is little difference between the new and the old, and no difference in their strength.

Thus the fears of those who believe that union can never be secure are groundless. It can be seen that it is not necessary for the ends to be in contact for them to unite. In the healing of a broken bone it is essential that the ends are kept in contact, if no shortening is to result from the pull of the muscles, and they must be carefully splinted in the correct position. It is the opposite with tendons, for the ends retract by the pull of the muscles, but the tendon sheath keeps them in the same longitudinal axis, so that the granulations sprouting from the ends must meet each other.

The rules proposed by Delpech for division of the Achilles tendon[5] hold good in general, and were endorsed and completed by Stromeyer:

(1) Only complete division of the tendon is effective.

(2) The skin immediately over the tendon must not be damaged; the incision should be as small as possible and well away from the tendon.

(3) After the operation the wound must be covered with a dressing to keep the air out.

(4) If the contracture is not relieved, search must be made for other shortened tendons, which must be divided in the same way, without damaging important structures.

(5) The after-care is, at first, rest, and then the long-continued use of a purpose-built splint to bring the limb into the required position.[6]

Experience has now shown that the results are better the earlier the splint is applied, and von Ammon and I have started immediately after the operation, without disturbing the healing.

CLUB-FOOT

This is not the place to discuss the aetiology of club-foot, except to say that it seems that the primary fault is arrested development of the bones

---

[5] J. M. Delpech, *De l'orthomorphie par rapport à l'espèce humaine,* Vol. 2, Paris, p. 321 (1828).

[6] L. Stromeyer, Die Durchschneidung der Achillessehne beim Klumpfusses, *Magazin ges. Heilk.* **39,** 195 (1832).

of the tarsus. It is not due to spasm of the calf muscles, for these are always relaxed, and, indeed, atrophied; the relatively common association of spina bifida with club-foot supports this. The shape of the bones is the main factor, and the tendons adapt to this faulty shape. Division of such tendons is beneficial, but it is easier to correct acquired deformities by tenotomy, where the bones go back to their normal position when the soft tissues are released.

The treatment of club-foot was for long the concern of orthopaedics, and operative surgery played no part, unless it was thought that it was better to have no foot than a deformed one, and it was amputated. Many splints were invented—some ingenious, but others ridiculous, heavy, clumsy, and expensive. Some patients abandoned the wearisome treatment half-way, and others came too late for treatment to be effective, or could not afford it. Many parents spared neither money nor trouble, and often paid out more in money than the weight of the child, to no avail. Splinting alone is only effective if started in early infancy, and continued for a long time. Tenotomy, however, can only overcome the obstacles that the soft tissues present to the cure of club-foot, and naturally the problems with the shape of the bones will remain.

Before dividing the Achilles tendon, the patient must be in good health. If there are any raw areas on the foot, the patient must rest until these are healed, or he will not be able to wear the splint. For the operation, he is laid on his belly, and the foot is held by two assistants to prevent involuntary movements. A stab incision, not more than a quarter of an inch long, is made two inches above the heel. Through this a narrow sickle-shaped bistoury is introduced, and turned towards the tendon, protecting the skin with the left hand. Very little force is needed for division of the tendon, which is recognized by a cracking sound; every fibre must be divided. Usually the foot can now be put into a reasonably normal position. If any other tendons are still tight, they are divided in the same way. The wound is covered with a small dressing, and the splint is immediately applied.

All surgeons now agree that there are no significant complications after this operation, so that both feet can be treated at the same time, except in older patients with very severe deformities.

WRYNECK

This may be due to curvature of the vertebrae, and division of the sternomastoid will not help. But even if the deformity started as a shortening of the muscle, the vertebrae become curved if the contracture has lasted for any length of time. There may also be asymmetry of the two sides of the head. Some surgeons have condemned operation, and they confine their treatment to massage with softening oils, strengthening the opposite side of the neck, and splinting the head in the correct position for a long time. In earlier times several surgeons divided the sterno-mastoid with good results. More recently Dupuytren has taken up the operation, dividing as much muscle as is necessary to straighten the head.[7] The muscle heals in the same way as tendon, and the same rules for operation apply. There is little danger; practice on the cadaver soon ensures that deeper structures are not injured. Dieffenbach has done this operation 30 times in the last few years with good results in all cases.

[7] F. A. von Ammon, *Parallele der französischen und deutschen Chirurgie*, Leipzig p. 374 (1823).

30

CONTRACTURE OF THE FINGERS

Permanent contracture of the fingers is not well known to German surgeons. According to Dupuytren it is due to shortening of the fascia in the hand;[1] other authors have suggested rheumatism, gout, trauma, fractures, or inflammation of the tendon sheaths. Dupuytren was the first to point out that it occurs mainly in people who do hard manual work. He cited a wine-merchant, who 'was obliged to perforate continually the casks with a gimlet', and a coachman, who 'had to ply his whip unceasingly on the backs of his jaded horses.'[2] It is common in masons and country people, who have to grip strongly with their hands. They first notice that they cannot fully extend their fingers, commonly the fourth, starting with the first phalanx, spreading to the other phalanges, and then to the two adjoining fingers. In the index finger only the first phalanx is involved; it can still move on the metacarpal, but even the heaviest weight will not extend it. When the ring finger is grossly contracted, the skin forms folds which are the result of its natural adhesion to the diseased tissue. At first glance it appears that the skin is the seat of the disease, but dissection shows that this is not so. When the fingers are contracted the patient can only carry out light tasks. If he grips strongly he gets pain, which disappears with rest, but returns on movement.

Many surgeons have thought that the cause lies in contracture and hardening of the skin, without realizing that the skin follows the contracture of the fascia. Others have suggested muscle spasm (but this is pure speculation for, with the exception of extension, all movements are free) or that the tendon sheaths or the joints are at fault. But most believe it to be a disease of the flexor tendons, and Dupuytren also thought this at first. But then he had the opportunity to do a post-mortem on a man with contracted fingers, whom he had kept under observation for a long time. After a drawing of the hand had been

[1] G. Dupuytren, *Leçons orales de clinique chirurgicale faites à l'Hôtel Dieu de Paris*, vol. 1 Paris, p. 1 (1832–34). [Baron Guillaume Dupuytren (1777–1835), Chief Surgeon at the Hôtel Dieu in Paris. See R. M. Goldwyn, *Plastic reconstr, Surg.* **42,** 194 (1968).]

[2] [G. Dupuytren, Permanent retraction of the fingers, produced by an affection of the palmar fascia, *Lancet* **2,** 222 (1833–34).]

made, the skin was removed from the palmar surface of the hand and fingers, and it immediately lost all its folds. Next the fascia was dissected, and Dupuytren found that it was contracted. Fibrous strands ran from its lower end to the sides of the affected fingers, and when he tried to extend these, the fascia became tighter. He then divided the bands to the fingers, and the contraction disappeared. The fingers were still a little flexed, and great force was needed to extend them completely. He found that the tendons and the joints were perfectly normal. It was clear that the deformity was due to contracture of the palmar aponeurosis, which must have arisen from contusion and long-continued strain.

The superficial palmar fascia is the expansion of the tendon of the palmaris brevis and of the anterior part of the annular ligament of the wrist. It has the function of holding the tendons together, and maintaining the concavity of the palm. At first very thick, it gradually becomes thinner, and ends at its lower border in four fibrous slips. These split to let the flexor tendons pass through, and are attached to the sides of the phalanges (not to the anterior surface, as most anatomists have thought). These are the bands which must be divided when they are contracted. The attachments of the skin to the aponeurosis make it difficult to separate them, and it is these attachments that account for the wrinkling of the skin. There is no danger to nerves or vessels in dividing the fascia, for it forms a sort of bridge over them, and protects them.

TREATMENT

The uncertainty about the origin of the disease naturally led to many different remedies. Some surgeons, including Astley Cooper, regarded it as incurable.[3] Dupuytren himself had tried steam, softening poultices, leeches, massage with mercury and calomel, alkaline douches, sulphur, and soaps at various temperatures. He had also used special extension apparatus without improvement, and had abandoned it because of the pain it caused. Some surgeons had recommended dividing the tendons, and this was carried out twice. In one of the cases there was inflammation of the tendon sheaths, and the patient nearly lost his life, but the finger remained bent. In the second case the effects were

[3] Cooper, Astley P., *A treatise on dislocations and on fractures of the joints,* London, p. 524 (1822). [Cooper distinguished between contraction of the theca and contraction of the aponeurosis, regarding the former as incurable, but recommending division of the band in the latter.]

not so severe, but the result was just as bad. As a result of his investigations, Dupuytren developed a new technique, with encouraging results.

Case-reports[4] In 1811 a wine-merchant was helping his men to move some casks, when he felt a cracking and a little pain in the palm of his left hand. For some time the hand was sensitive, but this gradually disappeared. He had almost forgotten the incident when he noticed that his ring finger was beginning to contract. Because there was no pain he did not pay much attention to this. But the disability increased year by year, and, by 1831, the fourth and fifth fingers were flexed into the palm. Several surgeons had advised him to have the tendons divided, but he came under the care of Dupuytren, who operated as follows:

The patient's hand was held firmly, and a transverse incision nearly an inch long was made over the metacarpo-phalangeal joint of the ring finger. The knife went first through the skin, and then, with an audible crack, through the palmar fascia, and immediately the finger could be straightened. To save the patient more pain, Dupuytren tried to divide the band to the little finger through the same incision, but this was not possible until two incisions were made in the finger, and another over the metacarpo-phalangeal joint. The little finger was now also completely free, and a splint was applied to the back of the hand to hold the fingers in extension.

Next day the pain was moderate, but there was some swelling due to the rather clumsy splint. This was replaced by a half-cylinder of pasteboard, to which four rods were attached, which could be lengthened or shortened, with rings on the ends to hold the tips of the fingers. At first the patient was more comfortable, but that evening the pain returned and the whole hand became swollen. Without removing the splint, Dupuytren ordered cold fomentations with lead lotion which gave relief. By the fifth day the swelling had abated, and suppuration was fully established. The extension of the fingers was increased. This extension-splinting delayed the healing of the wounds by pulling their edges apart. The incisions on the fingers healed more quickly than those in the palm. The patient wore the splint for a month, to keep the cut ends of the aponeurosis apart. When it was taken off he could bend his fingers, but there was a little stiffness which disappeared with exercise; he continued to wear the splint at night.

---

4 [See n. 2 above.]

Dupuytren did a similar operation on a 40-year-old coachman, whose fingers, mainly the ring, had been contracted for several years. The skin of the hand was in folds. When the finger was extended a band could be seen running from the finger into the palm. Both hands were similarly affected. The diagnosis was easy. Dupuytren made the patient move his fingers, and the contraction of the fascia could easily be seen. He made curved incisions, one at the base of the ring finger, and the other in the palm, in order to divide the extensions of the fascia. The finger immediately regained its normal mobility; bleeding was very slight. The operation on the other hand was postponed because the patient was exhausted. The after-care was the same as in the previous case.

Recently Goyrand has published his work on this subject, confirming Dupuytren's observations. But he thinks that a transverse incision leaves too big a raw surface, because it opens up when the finger is straightened. He advises that the skin should be incised longitudinally, and the fascia transversely. He notes that it is not only the third, fourth, and fifth fingers that are affected, because he has seen a case where the thumb was involved. He also contradicts the view that only hard manual work leads to the disease.[5] Although he and Dupuytren seem to have clarified the whole matter, some surgeons still insist that the flexor tendons can also be a cause of the disease.

Owing to lack of personal experience, and because so little is known about this subject in Germany, I have regarded it as essential to include this account. Dieffenbach has often carried out this operation successfully.

I have come to the end of my book well-aware that plastic surgery can still be improved in many ways. But I am also convinced that it will make ever more rapid strides towards perfection. I believe that I have given a full account of the position that it has now reached, 'but as nothing in the whole of medicine, or indeed in any activity, is unchanging, so this is not immutable.'[6]

---

5 G. Goyrand, Nouvelles recherches sur la rétraction permanente des doigts, *Mém. Acad. Méd. Paris* **3,** 489 (1834).

6 Tagliacozzi, *de curtorum*, Vol. 2, Chapter 13, p. 48.

BIBLIOGRAPHY

Account of the method of supplying Artificial noses; as practised by the natives of the Malabar Coast, *Philadelphia Medical Museum,* **2**, 343 (1806).

Adams, F., *The seven books of Paulus Aegineta*, for the Sydenham Society, London (1854).

Adams, W., *Practical observations on ectropium or the eversion of the eyelids, with the description of a new operation for the cure of that disease*, London (1812).

Ammon, F. A. von, *Parallele der französischen und deutschen Chirurgie*, Leipzig (1823).

Ammon, F. A. von, Beiträge zur Morioplastik, *Magazin ges. Heilk.* **32**, 162 (1830).

Ammon, F. A. von, *Das Symblepharon und die Heilung dieser Krankheit durch eine neue Operationsmethode,* 2nd edn, Dresden (1834).

Ammon, F. A. von, Dr. Dieffenbach's neue Methode der Blepharoplastik. Ein Sendschreiben an Dr. Fricke, *Z. Ophthal.* **4**, 428 (1835).

Ammon, F. A. von, *Commentatio chirurgica de physiologia tenotomiae experimentis illustrata,* Dresden (1837).

Ammon, F. A. von, Morioplastik, *Magazin ges. Heilk.* **39**, 173 (1837).

Amussat, J. Z., Observation sur une opération de vagin artificiel pratigée avec succès, par un nouveau procédé, suivie de quelques réflexions sur les vices de conformation du vagin, *Gaz. Méd.* p. 785 (1835).

Auria, V., *La Sicilia inventrice con li divertimenti geniali di Dr. Mongitore,* Palermo (1704).

Balfour, W., Two cases, with observations, demonstrative of the power of nature to reunite parts which have been, by accident, totally separated from the animal system, *Edinb. med. surg. J.* **10**, 421 (1814).

Baronio, G., *Degli innesti animali,* Milan (1804).

Barri, G., *De antiquitate et situ Calabriae,* Frankfurt (1600).

Baumgarten, M., *De chiloplastica et stomatopoësi*, Leipzig (1837).

Beck, C. J., Gelungener Fall einer Rhinoplastik, *Heidelb. klin. Annln.* **3**, 250, (1827).

Bellini, G., Colpodesmorafia, o sia suora operazione per la cura del prolasso della vagina come dell' utero, *Omod. Ann. univ.* **79**, 180 (1836).

Belmas, D.-G., *Recherches sur un moyen de déterminer des inflammations adhésives dans les cavités séreuses,* Paris (1829).

Benedetti, A., *Anatomiae sive historia corporis humani*, Venice (1502).

Benedict, T. W. G., *Beiträge zu den Erfahrungen über die Rhinoplastik nach der deutschen Methode*, Breslau (1828).

Bérard, A., Chute de la matrice, élytrorhaphie, *Gaz. Méd.* p. 541 (1835).
Berg, Chiloplastik, *Preuss. med. Verztg.* p. 251 (1836).
Bille, M., Nekrolog des Professor Dr. Eduard Zeis, *Sitzungsberichte der Gesellschaft für Natur- und Heilkunde zu Dresden*, **2**, 150 (1868–69).
Blandin, P. F., *Autoplastie ou restauration des parties du corps, qui ont été détruites à la faveur d'un emprunt fait à d'autres parties plus ou moins éloignées*, Paris (1836).
Blandin, P. F., Autoplastie faciale, *Bull. Acad. r. Méd.* **1**, 34 (1836).
Blasius, E., *Handbuch der Akiurgie*, Halle (1831).
Blasius, E., Neues Verfahren der Lippenbildung, *Z. Chir. Augenheilk.* **1**, 387 (1836).
Blegny, N. de, *Zodiacus medico-gallicus*, Geneva (1682).
Boinet, A.-A., Ectropion considérable suite de brûlure, blépharoplastie, procédé de M. Blandin, guérison, *Gaz. Méd.* p. 764 (1836).
Bossu, Sur la réunion de la troisiéme phalange du pouce après la section parfaite, *J. Méd. Pharm.* July, p. 78 (1770).
Boyer, A., Mémoire sur la meilleure forme des aiguilles propres à la réunion des plaies, *Mém. soc. méd. émul.* p. 97 (Paris, 1799).
Brach, B. Vorschlag zu einer neuen Operationsmethode des Entropiums, *Preuss. med. Vertztg.* p. 27 (1837).
Braun, J. A., Wiederanheilung eines gänzlich abgeschnittenen Fingers, *Magazin ges. Heilk.* **14**, 112 (1823).
Bünger, H. C., Gelungener Versuch einer Nasenbildung aus einem völlig getrennten Hautstück aus dem Beine, *J. Chir. Augenheilk.* **4**, 569 (1823).
Bushnan, J. S., *Surgical observations on the restoration of the nose*, London (1833).
Butler, S., *Hudibras*, London (1710).

Cambrelin, Chéiléoplastie, *Archs gén. Méd.* **26**, 263 (1831).
Carpue, J. C., *An account of two successful operations for restoring a lost nose from the integuments of the forehead in the cases of two officers of His Majesty's Army*, London (1816).
Carron du Villards, C.-J., Restauration des paupières, *Gaz. Hôp. Paris* p. 8 (1836).
Celsus, A. C. *de medicina*, Book 7, Chapters 9, 25.
Chelius, M. J., Gelungene Lippen- und Nasenbildung an demselben Subjecte, *Heidelb. klin. Annln.* **6**, 523 (1830).
Chelius, M. J., *Handbuch der Chirurgie*, Heidelberg (1834).
Clot-Bey, A.-B., *Histoire d'une tumeur éléphantiaque du scrotum du poids de 110 livres, extirpée avec succès chez un Arabe*, Marseilles (1830).
Clot-Bey, A.-B., Observation d'une tumeur éléphantiaque du scrotum de 50 livres, extirpée avec succès, *Gaz. Hôp. Paris* p. 488 (1833).
Collier, Heilung eines künstlichen Afters durch Hautüberpflanzung, *J. Chir. Augenheilk.* **2**, 655 (1821).
Cooper, A. P., *A treatise on dislocations and on fractures of the joints*, London (1822).
Cooper, A. P., and Travers, B., *Surgical essays*, London (1818–19).
Coronelli, V. *Biblioteca universale*, Venice (1706).

Cortesi, G. B., *Miscellaneorum medicinalium decades denae*, Messina (1625).

Davies, J., A case where the Taliacotian operation was successfully performed, *Lond. med. Repos.* **21**, 39 (1824).

Delpech, J. M., *Chirurgie clinique de Montpellier*, Paris (1828).

Delpech, J. M., Observation d'un cas d'intumescence énorme du scrotum, symptome d'éléphantiasis, *Chirurgie clinique de Montpellier*, **2**, 5 (Paris, 1828).

Delpech, J. M., *De l'orthomorphie par rapport à l'espéce humaine*, Paris (1828).

Dieffenbach, J. F., Transplantationensversuche bei Thieren, *J. Chir. Augenheilk.* **6**, 122 (1824).

Dieffenbach, J. F., Ueberpflanzung völlig getrennter Hautstücke bei einer Frau und Wiederanheilung einer grösstentheils abgehauenen Wange, *J. Chir. Augenheilk.* **6**, 482 (1824).

Dieffenbach, J. F., Die abgeänderte umschlungene Nath als schnelles Heilmittel bei Gesichtswunden, *Annln. ges. Heilk.* **8**, 129 (1827).

Dieffenbach, J. F., Neue Methode der Lippenbildung, *Magazin ges. Heilk.* **25**, 383 (1827).

Dieffenbach, J. F., *Chirurgische Erfahrungen, besonders über die Wiederherstellung zerstörter Theile des menschlichen Körpers nach neuen Methoden*, Berlin, (1829–34).

Dieffenbach, J. F., Heilung eines schwierigen Falles von künstlichem After durch einen Lanzenstich hervorgebracht, nach einer neue Methode, *Caspers Wschr.* p. 265 (1834).

Dieffenbach, J. F., Einige Bemerkungen aus und über Paris. Ueber einen Fall von Blepharoplastik, *Caspers Wschr.* p. 8 (1835).

Dieffenbach, J. F., Ueber Mutterkränze und Radicalcur des Scheiden- und Gebärmuttervorfalles, *Preuss. med. Verztg.* p. 151 (1836).

Dieffenbach, J. F., Ueber die Heilung der Blasen-Scheiden-Fisteln und Zerreissungen der Blase und Scheide, *Preuss. med. Verztg.* pp. 117, 173 (1836).

Dieffenbach, J. F., Ueber die Heilung widernatürlicher Oeffnungen in dem vordern Theile der Harnröhre nach neuen Methoden, *Z. ges. med.* **2**, 1 (1836).

Dieffenbach, J. F., *Die Operative Chirurgie*, Vol. 1, Leipzig (1845).

Dionis, P., *Cours d'opérations de chirurgie*, Brussels, (1708).

Dreyer, J. T., *Nova blepharoplastices methodus*, Diss., Vienna (1831).

Du Hamel, H. L., Recherches sur la réunion des plaies des arbres, sur la façon dont la greffe s'unit au sujet sur lequel on l'applique, sur la réunion des plaies des animaux, et quelques exemples de greffes appliquées sur des animaux, *Hist. Acad. r. Sci.* année 1746, p. 319 (Paris, 1751).

Dupuytren, G., Operations for the removal of various deformities at the Hospital of Lyons, *Lond. med. Gaz.*, **5**, 799 (1830).

Dupuytren, G., Chéiléoplastie, pratiquée avec succès, *Gaz. Hôp. Paris* p. 273 (1830).

Dupuytren, G., *Leçons orales de clinique chirurgicale, faites à l'Hôtel Dieu de Paris*, Paris (1832).

Dupuytren, G., Permanent retraction of the fingers, produced by an affection of the palmar fascia, *Lancet* **2**, 222 (1833–34).

Dutrochet, H., *Gaz. Santé, Paris,* no. 9 (1817).

Dybeck, A. F., Glücklich ausgeführter Ersatz eines Nasenflügels, *J. Chir. Augenheilk.* **5**, 364 (1823).

Dzondi, C. H., *Beiträge zur Vervollkommnung der Heilkunde,* Halle (1816).

Dzondi, C. H., *Kurze Geschichte des klinischen Institutes,* Halle, (1818).

Dzondi, C. H., Bildung eines neuen unteren Augenlides aus der Wange, *J. prakt. heilk.* **47**, 99 (1818).

Dzondi, C. H., Ersatz des linken Nasenflügels. Transplantation aus der Haut eines andern Individui, *Magazin ges. Heilk.* **6**, 1 (1819)

Eloy, N. F. J., *Dictionnaire historique de médecine ancienne et moderne,* Mons (1778).

Fabry von Hilden, W., *Opera quae exstant omnia,* Frankfurt (1646).

Fauchard, P., *Le chirurgien dentiste, ou traité des dents,* Paris (1728).

Fazio, B., *De viris illustribus liber,* Florence (1745).

Fergusson, W., Case of reparation of the nose, *Edinb. med. surg. J.* **43**, 363 (1835).

Feyens, T., *de praecipuis artis chirurgicae controversiis,* Frankfurt (1649).

Finck, Ph., *Ueber radicale Heilung reponibler Brüche,* Freiburg (1837).

Fioravanti, L., *Tesoro della vita humana,* Venice (1673).

Fludd, R., *Defense of weapon-salve or the squeezing of parson Foster's spunge,* London (1635).

Franco, P., *Traité des hernies contenant une ample déclaration de toutes leurs espèces et autres excellentes parties de la chirurgie,* Lyons (1561).

Fricke, J. C. G., *Die Bildung neuer Augenlider (Blepharoplastik) nach Zerstörungen,* Hamburg (1829).

Fricke, J. C. G., Die Episiorhaphie bei Vorfällen der Mutterscheide und Gebärmutter, *Annalen der chirurgischen Abtheilung des allgemeinen Krankenhauses in Hamburg* **2**, (1833) 142.

Fricke, J. C. G., Wiederersatz des knorpeligen Theiles eines gänzlich zerstörten Septum narium aus der Oberlippe, *J. Chir. Augenheilk.* **22**, 456 (1834).

Galen, C. *Methodus medendi*, Book 14, Chapter 16, editio Kühniana, Leipzig (1827).

Garanne, R. de la, Sur la réparation de quelques parties du corps humains mutilées, *Hist. Acad. r. Sci.* **4**, 32 (1721).

Garengeot, R. J. C., *Traité des opérations de chirurgie*, Paris (1731).

Gentleman's Magazine **64**, 891 (1794).

Gibson, T., Delpech: his contributions to plastic surgery and the astonishing case of scrotal elephantiasis, *Br. J. plast. Surg.* **9**, 4 (1956).

Gibson, T., Eduard Zeis (1807–1868) plastic surgical bibliographer extraordinary, *Br. J. plast. Surg.* **29**, 277 (1976).

Gnudi, M. T. and Webster, J. P., *The life and times of Gaspare Tagliacozzi, surgeon of Bologna (1545–1599)*, New York (1950).

Goldwyn, R. M., Johann Friedrich Dieffenbach (1794–1847), *Plastic reconstr. Surg.* **42**, 18 (1968).

Goldwyn, R. M., Guillaume Dupuytren, *Plastic reconstr. Surg.* **42**, 194 (1968).

Gourmelenus, Stephanus, *Chirurgicae artis*, Paris (1580).

Goyrand, G., Nouvelles recherches sur la rétraction permanente des doigts, *Mém. Acad. Méd. Paris* **3**, 489 (1834).

Gräfe, C. F. von, *Rhinoplastik, oder die Kunst den Verlust der Nase organisch zu ersetzen,* Berlin (1818).

Gräfe, C. F. von, Gräfe misslangen alle (bis 1821) an Menschen und Thieren gemachten Versuch zur Transplantation ganz getrennter Theile, *J. Chir. Augenheilk.* **2**, 1 (1821).

Gräfe, C. F. von, Meloplastik, *J. Chir. Augenheilk.* **2**, 14 (1821).

Gräfe, C. F. von, Neue Beiträge zur Kunst Theile des Angesichts organisch zu ersetzen, *J. Chir. Augenheilk.* **2**, 27 (1821).

Gräfe, C. F. von, Fall von Rhinoplastik aus der Stirn, *J. Chir. Augenheilk.* **12**, 11 (1828).

Gräfe, C. F. von, Fall von Rhinoplastik, *J. Chir. Augenheilk.* **13**, 2 (1829).

Gräfe, C. F. von, Organischer Ersatz der Nase aus der Armhaut, *J. Chir. Augenheilk.* **22**, 8 (1834).

Graham, Maria, *Letters on India,* London (1814).

Hall, Marshall, Case of prolapsus uteri cured by a new operation, *Lond. med. Gaz.* **9**, 269 (1832).

Heidenreich, F. W., Heilung eines Krebses an der Nase mit vollständiger Herstellung der Gestalt und Farbe, *J. Chir. Augenheilk.* **20**, 456 (1833).

Heister, L., *Institutiones chirurgicae,* Amsterdam (1750).

Helmont, J. B. van, *Opera omnia*, Frankfurt (1682).

Hicrarrah or Madras Gazette, 5 August 1794.

Hoffacker, G. W., Beobachtungen über die Anheilung abgehauener Stücke der Nase und Lippen, *Heidelb. klin. Annln.* **4**, 232 (1828).

Höfft, S. F., Rhinoplastices Britannicae seu Nasi restituti ope insiti a fronte ademti corii specimen, *Commentationes soc. phys.-med. apud univ. liter. Caes. Mossquensem instit.* **3**, 33 (1823).

Hunter, J., *The natural history of the teeth,* London (1771).

Hutchison, A. C., Case in which the nasal operation has been recently performed, *Edinb. med. surg. J.* **14**, 344 (1818).

Ireland, Case of procidentia uteri successfully treated by operation, *Dubl. J. med. chem. Sci.* **6**, 484 (1835).

Jameson, G., On the permanent cure of femoral hernia, *Lancet* **2**, 142 (1829–30).

Jessen, J. von, *Institutiones chirurgicae*, Wittenberg (1601).

Jobert, A.-J., Cancer de la paupière inférieure droite, extirpation, blépharoplastie, guérison, *Gaz. Méd.* p. 404 (1835).
Jobert, A.-J., [Case demonstration], *Gaz. Méd.* p. 76 (1836).
Jobert, A.-J., Sur les fistules vesico-vaginales *Gaz. Méd.* p. 145 (1836).
Jüngken, J. C., *Die Lehre von den Augenoperationen*, Berlin (1829).

Kaufmann, K.-F., *Die ersten 100 Jahre Chirurgie in Marburg*, Diss., Marburg (1963).
Klein, K. C. von, Hingeworfene chirurg. Bruchstücke, *Heidelb. klin. Annln.* **2**, 103 (1826).
Koch, L., Ein Beitrag zur Episiorhaphie, *J. Chir. Augenheilk.* **25**, 667 (1837).
Krüger-Hansen, B. K., Practische Reminiscenzen, *J. Chir. Augenheilk.* **4**, 543. (1822).

Labat, P. A. L., *De la rhinoplastie, art de restaurer ou de refaire complètement le nez*, Paris (1834).
Lallemand, C.-F., Plaie à la face avec perte de substance, guérie par l'application d'un lambeau détaché des parties voisines, *Archs gén. Méd.* **6**, 242 (1824).
Lancet **1**, 385 (1834–5).
Lanfranc of Milan, *Chirurgia Magna.* In *Collectio Veneta*, Venice (1519).
Larrey, D. J., *Clinique chirurgicale*, Paris (1829).
Lawrence, W., Nature and treatment of injuries, *Lancet* **1**, 521 (1829–30).
Lespagnol, N. L., Observation sur la réunion immédiate de l'extrémité d'un doigt qui avoit été entièrement coupée et separée du corps, *J. Méd. Pharm.* **39**, 273 (1817).
Lisfranc, J., Mémoire sur la rhinoplastie, *Bull. Sci. méd.* **12**, 238 (1827).
Liston, R., Operation for restoring the columna nasi, *Edinb. med. surg. J.* **35**, 84 (1831).
Lond. med. Gaz. **5**, 799 (1830).
Loubet, J. A. , *Traité des playes d'armes à feu*, Paris (1753).
Lynn, W. In C. Bell, *Institutes of surgery*, Vol. 1, Edinburgh, p. 226 (1838).

Maisonabe, C. A., *Clinique sur les difformités dans l'espèce humaine*, Paris (1834).
Malgaigne, J. F., *Manuel de médecine opératoire*, Brussels (1834).
Markiewicz, R., Nachricht über die Anheilung einer zwei Stunden lang völlig abgetrennten Nase, *J. Chir. Augenheilk.* **7**, 538 (1825).
Martinet de la Creuse, Mémoire sur un nouveau procédé opératoire à prévenir la récidive du cancer, *Gaz. Méd.* p. 657 (1834).
May, H., Successful attempt of reconstruction of a nose from a completely separated piece of skin from the leg, *Plastic reconstr. Surg.* **44**, 569 (1969).
Meek'ren, J. van, *Observationes medico-chirurgicae,* Amsterdam (1682).
Memoir of Baron Graefe, *Lancet* **1**, 969 (1833–34).
Mercuriale, H., *de decoratione,* Frankfurt (1587).
Merrem, D. C. T., *Animadversiones quaedam chirurgicae experimentis in animalibus factis*, Giessen (1810).

Michaelis, H. S., Ueber die Schwächung der Sehnen durch Einschneidung, *J. prakt. Arzneik. Wundarzneik.* **23**, 1 (1811).
Michaelis, H. S., *Geschichte zweier gelungenen Fälle, wo der Verlust der Nase vermittelst der Stirnhaut ersetzt wurde*, Berlin (1817).
Minding, J., Ein Beitrag zur Chirurgia curtorum. In Clarus, J. C. A. und Radius, J., *Beiträge zur praktische Heilkunde*, Vol. 3, Leipzig, p. 194 (1836).
Molinetti, A., *Dissertationes anatomico-pathologicae*, Venice (1675).
Montégre, A.-F.-J., *Gaz. Santé, Paris*, no. 7 (1817).
Mütter, T. D., *Cases of autoplastic*, Philadelphia (1838).

Nasal operation, *Lancet* **1**, 233 (1823).
Nichet, J. P., Coup de feu à la face, perforation du plancher de la bouche, autoplastie, guérison, *Gaz. Méd.* p. 454 (1836).

On plastic surgery, *Br. for. med. Rev.* **7**, 386, 392, 393, 408, 416 (1839).
On plastic surgery, *Br. for. med. Rev.* **19**, 398 (1846).
On the development of adhesions of serous membranes, and their application to several surgical diseases, *Br. for med. Rev.* **6**, 232 (1838).
On the radical cure of hernia, *Br. for. med. Rev.* **6**, 341 (1838).

Paré, A., *Opera chirurgica*, Frankfurt (1594).
Paul of Aegina, *opera*, Leyden (1589).
Pennant, T., *The view of Hindoostan*, London (1798).
Percy, P.-F., *Dictionaire des sciences médicales*, Vol. 12, Paris, p. 343 (1815).
Percy, P.-F., and Laurent, C., *Dictionaire des sciences médicales*, Vol. 36, Paris, p. 74 (1819).
Peters, E. O., *De blepharoplastice*, Diss., Leipzig (1836).
Petit, J. L., *Oeuvres complétes (bibliothéque chirurgicale)*, Limoges (1837).
Phillips, C., Restoration of the nose and eyelid, *Lancet* **1**, 182 (1834–5).
Plath, Geschichte einer Geburt nach gemachter Episiorhaphie, *Z. ges med.* **2**, 442 (1836).

Read, A., *Chirurgorum comes, or the whole practice of chirurgery*, London (1687).
Rhinoplastic operation performed by M. Lisfranc, followed by Death, *Lancet* **2**, 808 (1827–8).
Riberi, A., Fall von Lippenbildung, *Repert. med. chir. Piemonte* (Oct. 1834).
Richerand, A.-B., *Nosographie et thérapeutique chirugicales*, 5th edn, Paris (1821).
Richter, A. G., *Anfangsgründen der Wundarzneikunst*, 3rd edn, Göttingen (1802).
Rogers, B. O., Carl Ferdinand von Graefe (1787–1840), *Plastic reconstr. Surg.* **46**, 554 (1970).
Rost, G., *De chilo- et stomatoplastice*, Diss., Berlin (1836).
Rudtorffer, F. X., *Abhandlung über die einfachste und sicherste Operationsmethode eingesperrter Leisten- und Schenkelbrüche*, Vienna (1808).
Ruppius, J. K., Eine Rhinoplastik aus der Stirnhaut, *Z. ges. med.* **4**, 243 (1837).

Rust, J. N., Neue Methode verstümmelte und durchbrochene Nasen auszubessern. Ein Beitrag zur Geschichte der Nasenrestaurationen, *Magazin ges. Heilk.* **2**, 351 (1817).

Saad, M. N. and Barron, J. N., Ambroise Paré. His contributions to plastic surgery, *Plastic reconstr. Surg.* **46**, 271 (1970).

Sancassani, D. A., *Dilucidazioni fisico-mediche,* Rome (1731).

Schenk von Grafenberg, J., *Observationum medicarum,* Frankfurt (1609).

Schwerdt, F. R. T., *Die Gaumennaht,* Berlin (1829).

Seerig, W., Fall von Elephantiasis scroti *Magazin ges. Heilk.* **47**, 119 (1836).

Serre, M., Nouveau procédé de chéiloplastie, *Gaz. Méd.* p. 238 (1835).

Sick, R., Ueber einige durch Armhautüberpflanzungen zu Berlin, Breslau und Wilna gemachte rhinoplastische Operationen. *J. Chir. Augenheilk.* **12**, 630 (1828).

Sprengel, K., *Geschichte der Chirurgie,* Halle (1819).

Staub, J., *De blepharoplastice,* Diss., Berlin (1835).

Stromeyer, L., Die Durchschneidung der Achillessehne beim Klumpfusses, *Magazin ges. Heilk.* **39**, 195 (1832).

Svitzer, E., *Beretnig om nogle Forsog til at danne en ny Forhud. Bibliothek for Laeger, Udgivet af Directionen,* Vol. 5, Copenhagen, p. 40 (1831).

Syme, J., Praeternatural aperture in the nose. Closure by transplanting a flap of skin, *Edinb. med. surg. J.* **44**, 5 (1835).

Tagliacozzi, Gaspare., *de curtorum chirurgia per insitionem,* 2 Vols, Venice (1597).

Taliacotian operation for a new nose, *Lancet* **4**, 21, 159 (1823–4).

The Tatler **4**, 313 (1710).

Tax, C., *De septi narium restitutione,* Diss., Berlin (1836).

Textor, K., Rhinoplastik aus der Stirnhaut nach der indischen Methode, *J. Chir. Augenheilk.* **6**, 374 (1824).

Textor, K., Ueber Chiloplastik, *Isis* **21**, 496 (1828).

Thomson, J., *Lectures on inflammation,* Edinburgh (1813).

Tyrell, F., A case of loss of nose, and restoration by the Taliacotian operation, *Lond. med. surg. J.* **6**, 730 (1835).

Velpeau, A. L. M., *Nouveaux éléments de médecine opératoire,* Paris (1832).

Velpeau, A. L. M., Fistule laryngienne traitée avec succès, au moyen d'une opération nouvelle, *Gaz. Hôp. Paris* p. 209 (1832).

Vesalius, A. *Chirurgiae magnae,* Leyden (1725).

Walther, P. F. von, Wiederanheilung der bei der Trepanation ausgebohrten Knochenscheibe, *J. Chir. Augenheilk.* **2**, 571 (1821).

Walther, P. F. von, Wiederanheilung einer ganz abgehauenen Nase, *J. Chir. Augenheilk.* **7**, pp. 521, 530 (1825).

Warren, J. M., Rhinoplastic operation, *Boston med. surg. J.* **16**, 69 (1837).

Wells, T. S., Practical essays on plastic surgery, *Med. Times and Gaz.* **9**, 9 (1854).

Werneck, W., Ueber die künstliche Mundwinkel- und Lippenbildung durch blütige Umschlagung der Mundschleimhaut, *J. Chir. Augenheilk.* **14**, 202 (1830).

Wiesmann, J. H. F., *De coalitu partium a reliquo corpore prorsus disjunctarum*, Leipzig (1824).

Zeis, E., Heilung eines Loches im weichen Gaumen, welche nach mehren vergeblichen Versuchen der Staphyloraphie zuletzt durch Anlegung von Seitenaperturen ohne Nähte bewirkt ward, *J. Chir. Augenheilk.* **25**, 495 (1837).

Zeis, E., *Drei chirurgische Abhandlungen über die plastische Chirurgie des Celsus*, Dresden and Leipzig (1843).

Zeis, E., *Die Literatur und Geschichte der plastischen Chirurgie*, Leipzig (1863); and *Nachträge dazu*, Leipzig (1864). English translation: T. J. S. Patterson, *The Zeis index and history of plastic surgery*, The McDowell Series of Plastic Surgical Indexes, Vol. 1, Williams and Wilkins, Baltimore (1977).

INDEX